AIDS: THE WOMEN

Edited by
INES RIEDER and PATRICIA RUPPELT

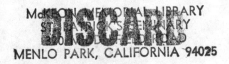
Cleis Press
SAN FRANCISCO • PITTSBURGH

Published in the United States by Cleis Press, P.O. Box 8933, Pittsburgh, Pennsylvania 15221, and P.O. Box 14684, San Francisco, California 94114.

Printed in the United States.
Cover and text design: Pete Ivey
Cover Photograph: Gipsy Ray
Typesetting: Sunita Vatuk/CalGraphics

Hedwig Bönsch's article is excerpted by permission of the author from *Die Schwester/Der Pfleger*, October 1987.

Library of Congress Cataloging-in-Publication Data

AIDS : the women / edited by Ines Rieder and Patricia Ruppelt. — 1st ed.
        p.   cm.
    Bibliography: p.

    1. AIDS (Disease)—Social aspects. 2. Women—Diseases.
I. Rieder, Ines, 1954- . II. Ruppelt, Patricia, 1956- .
RC607.A26A3645 1988
362.1'9697'92—dc19   88-28561
                                                            CIP

015128

Notes & Acknowledgments

M OST AUTHORS in this anthology have used their real names. Some have chosen to use only their initials, or, in some cases, have decided to write under a pseudonym. References to other people sometimes include real names, and sometimes not. We have not identified which names are real and which fictitious.

The selections by Ute Phielepeit, Erika Parsa and Hedwig Bönsch were originally written in German and translated by Ines Rieder. The selections by Margareth, Mônica Pita, and Silvia Ramos were originally written in Brazilian Portuguese and translated by Ines Rieder and Marlene Rodrigues.

For definitions of AIDS-related medical terms in each article, please refer to the glossary. For more detailed information, we advise you to consult some of the excellent brochures put out by the San Francisco AIDS Foundation and the New York Gay Men's Health Crisis. For more detailed information on these and other AIDS-related organizations, please check the resource list.

Above all we would like to thank all the contributors whether or not their stories were included. We also would like to thank all those who helped us find possible authors, develop ideas, edit and proofread drafts and especially those who listened. Here we name only a few: Anju Gurnani, Marlene Rodrigues and all her Brazilian friends, Merle Shore, Nicole Ravenel, Adelheid Zöfel, Erika Parsa, Annemarie Schurzmann, Teresa Fusillo-Henkel, Verena Baustädter, Ute Phielepeit, Linda Fogel, Sandy Chelnov, Alan Snitow, Arthur Squires, Jill Hannum, Sandra Meucci, Cecilia Brunazzi, Andrea Pearlstein, Donna Scism, Reyna Cowan, Lisa Capalidini, the women from *Connexions* magazine, Ruth Schwartz, Catherine Maier, Rick Garfunkel, Denise Ribble.

Thanks to Frédérique Delacoste and Felice Newman of Cleis Press for their patience, their work and their belief that this project could actually turn into a viable anthology.

Contents

Introduction

A Bittersweet Dance

"All pain is shattering; but when it's shared, at least it is no longer a banishment. It is not out of morose delectation, nor out of exhibitionism, nor out of provocation that writers often tell of hideous or deeply saddening experiences: through the medium of words they render these experiences universal and allow their readers, deep in their private unhappiness, to know the consolation of sisterhood. In my opinion one of the essential functions of literature, a function which means that nothing else can take its place, is the overcoming of that isolation which is common to us all and which nevertheless makes us strangers to each other."
— *Simone de Beauvoir*

Sickness and death are two elements of life which all of us have to confront at any given moment. Even though these are realities nobody can escape, we attempt to carry on the comfortable mystification that they will not happen to us, but only to others. And these others are removed as far as possible from our day-to-day concerns. Then one day it hits. If it happens to be cancer or a car accident, or something else that we have gotten accustomed to, there is a set of prepared consolations to reduce our grief.

AIDS took everybody by surprise — at least those living in the so-called developed countries, where epidemics are rarely heard of, and where, if they occur, societies are quick to deal with them. Having grown up in one of these societies, and having incorporated its values and beliefs, I found it very hard to accept the fact that Michael, one of my best friends, had AIDS. When he began worrying about his health and some AIDS-related symptoms started to appear, I refused to see them.

Then reality caught up with us. It was the spring of 1986; he was living in Paris and had been diagnosed with AIDS. I was preparing to leave Brazil, where I had been living for the last two years, and I was on my way to spend some time in Portugal. But my friends in Paris informed me of his worsening condition, and in no time I was at his bedside twenty-four hours a day for three months. In June 1986, I saw his ashes fly back to his beloved/hated Alabama.

It took me almost two years to absorb the fact that he was dead. It

9

took me the same amount of time to understand that this tragedy had fallen upon him, and as consequence upon his lover, his family, and his friends. It took several months of writing to clarify my relationship with Michael's life and dying. It took getting involved in editing this anthology to put my own experience into a larger context.

Sitting here and reading all these personal accounts of women who went through similar experiences, I see in each piece some of my own reflections. If nothing else, at least it gives me an idea of my own dimensions as a human being, of my fears, my strengths, my illusions. It reminds me that I am neither a coward nor a Mother Teresa, but just a human being passionately involved with life, wanting to protect herself against death and disease, but also willing to face death and to dance with it the bittersweet song of our existence.

Ines Rieder
Oakland, California
July 1988

From the Outside In

INITIALLY MY INTEREST in this project had more to do with its format and its focus on a women's issue than on the subject of AIDS itself. For many years, I have worked in alternative media, exploring issues important to women's lives. I approach these concerns through the writings and testimonies of women, since their words yield a certain depth and honesty absent in an impersonal approach.

Working on this anthology was my first step into the world of AIDS. Living in the San Francisco Bay Area, I was certainly aware of the epidemic. But since it had not entered my immediate circle of friends and family, I kept my distance, as if that would protect me from its harm. I had been touched by accounts of people with AIDS and enraged at the discrimination and bigotry they had to face; yet, I maintained a sense of being separate from it.

As I learned a few basic statistics — for instance, that the major cause of death for women between the ages of 25 and 34 in New York City is AIDS — I woke up to the magnitude of this problem. It was not only this information itself that I found compelling, but the fact that I had been so unaware of the dimensions of the problem.

The immediacy of the epidemic did not allow me to remain on its outskirts for long. I remember my first Women's AIDS Network meeting. About three dozen women were working through a crowded agenda of policy decisions regarding women and AIDS, and swapping information about their own work, resources, suggestions for funding and requests for help with projects. They approached their work with a sense of urgency that I hadn't experienced previously. I could imagine this group crowded together on a steep slope, slowing the progress of a large boulder. The enormity of the issues regarding women and AIDS became clear to me then.

The striking diversity of women affected by AIDS was brought home to me at a party I attended for the members of a support group for HIV-positive women, as well as for women involved with AIDS work and women with AIDS. I looked around at this group and realized that I had never been in one room with people representing such a variety of social and ethnic backgrounds — young lawyers, a grandmother, an ex-prostitute AIDS educator, social workers, ex-IV drug users, feminist psychoanalysts, lesbians and heterosexual women. Similarly, working on this project I met many women living under very different circumstances. One week I would be at the San Francisco ballet discussing the effect of AIDS on the workplace of a prima ballerina. The next week I would be a few blocks away in the economically depressed Tenderloin district speaking with a woman with AIDS.

After working on this anthology for a couple of months, receiving daily in my mailbox submissions of personal stories full of pain and growth, and after long conversations with women whose lives had been changed by their involvement with the epidemic, I realized that I, too, had acquired the zealous attitude that seems to exude from many in the AIDS world. I found that some of my friends shied away from discussions about my work, to some degree mirroring the distance I had formerly felt toward this issue. I gravitated toward acquaintances who could understand my own increasing level of involvement with AIDS.

Once the bulk of the work on the project was completed, I traveled to India. Since India has relatively few reported cases, I expected a welcome break from my immersion in the subject of AIDS. However, from my first day in that country, I realized I couldn't escape the realities of the pandemic. The moralistic director of the prestigious Indian Council for Medical Research was spearheading legislation banning sex with foreigners as a policy to prevent the spread of AIDS. One of the more extreme examples of the sensationalized coverage of AIDS in the mainstream media was the photo of a prostitute who had allegedly died of AIDS being put into a body bag at the morgue. Soon I was clipping articles and making plans to send information about AIDS from U.S. prostitutes' rights organizations to Indian women's groups upon my return.

As the anthology is on its way to the printer, I am left wondering what my next step will be. After gaining a lot of knowledge and experience related to AIDS, in what ways will I be involved in the future? So many distinct images pass through my mind while contemplating the possibilities: health and social service workers in a heated discussion of the policies and practices of mandatory testing; the physical and emotional exhaustion of a woman whose close companion recently died of AIDS; a medical researcher clicking off facts and statistics about the epidemic; a woman on television explaining her initial HIV infection symptoms.

Whatever the next phase of my involvement, I am definitely no longer an outsider to this epidemic. Looking back, I can see that fear and ignorance fueled my desire to maintain a distance from AIDS. By perpetuating this illusion, I was at the greatest risk for both the physical and the political dangers of AIDS. I hope that by reading this book more people will be encouraged to realize their own connection to the epidemic, and integrate this understanding into their personal and work lives.

Patricia Ruppelt
Oakland, California
August 1988

AIDS Realities and Facts

THE PURPOSE OF this anthology is to give a face, or many faces, to women's involvement and affliction with the AIDS epidemic. Each contribution is from a woman whose personal or work life has been directly affected and changed by AIDS; each is unique in its style and perspective. Each of these stories is based on reality or real events, thus documenting women's roles in the AIDS epidemic.

Most of the women whose voices we hear are from the United States and Western Europe; some are from Brazil, and there is one contribution each from Zimbabwe and the Philippines. Until recently in the United States and Europe, AIDS has been portrayed as a disease of gay men. It continues to be perceived this way, even though a large and ever-increasing number of IV drug users — male and female — has come down with AIDS. There has been little talk about the many women in several African countries who have been diagnosed with AIDS, a fate that is now shared by women here in the United States and in Western Europe.

This book allows us to glimpse the everyday realities of women who have tested positive for HIV or who have developed AIDS-related symptoms. We have put all these stories together without distinguishing between people who are HIV-positive and those who have ARC or AIDS symptoms.

The daily news and new scientific findings make it difficult to consider this project done. We are in the middle of the AIDS epidemic — and most of these stories don't have an ending. But the stories' content — with all their emotions, compassion and pain — remain unchanged. The authors have focused on these human aspects rather than the complex medical world surrounding AIDS or the fast-changing facts.

The worldwide AIDS epidemic is a crisis. Countries with a somewhat adequate health care and social welfare system have so far managed to extend these services to people with AIDS. The governments and administrations in those countries where such an infrastructure is nonexistent or poorly developed, including the United States, have been challenged by this epidemic. In the United States, talk about an extensive national health care plan and a humane welfare system are once again brought in sharper focus, and there is an increasing demand and pressure for change.

The high level of involvement of those working in AIDS organizations and providing services for people with AIDS and AIDS-related problems is impressive. They project a strong sense of urgency and duty in regard to their work. Many contributors to this book use the metaphor of fighting a war to describe their work "on the front lines" of AIDS.

The effects of AIDS on their personal lives have changed the perspectives of our contributors and the people around them. AIDS brings with it many trials, including those of dealing with a life-threatening disease. The women presented in this anthology describe just this — how the challenge of AIDS has changed their perceptions of their work and of themselves.

Since this pandemic and this anthology go beyond the shores of the United States, it is essential to give a brief overview of the international situation regarding AIDS. As of July 1988, 108,176 people from 137 countries have been reported as having AIDS. The World Health Organization (WHO), the official record keeper, estimates that the number of cases might be at least double that, since many cases go unreported. It also speculates that about 10 million people worldwide may be HIV-infected. Unfortunately WHO statistics are not gender specific. Some of the contributions in this anthology give specific facts about women with AIDS for the regions or countries that they discuss.

When looking at the numbers of reported AIDS cases internationally, it is important to keep in mind the disparity in national resources available for health care and disease monitoring. With the exception of the U.S. figures, which are taken from the Centers for Disease Control (CDC), the following statistics are from WHO reports, while most of the annotated comments are based on information supplied by the Panos Institute's dossier, *AIDS in the Third World*.

North America

The CDC has reported cases of women with AIDS in the United States since April 1984, including categorization of cases by gender and means of transmission. As of July 1988, 68 percent of the U.S. cases are among gay or bisexual men with no IV drug history. Blacks make up 26 percent of the reported AIDS cases, and Latinos 15 percent.

15

Women compose about 9 percent of the 67,273 cases reported. Between January and July 1988, women made up 11 percent of the total number of new cases. Of the 4,870 cases of women and girls with AIDS, 51 percent are black, 28 percent are white and 20 percent are Latinas. Given that blacks make up 12 percent and Latinos 7 percent of the general population, these figures show the disproportionate effect of AIDS on people of color.

More than half of the reported cases of women with AIDS in the United States are linked to IV drug use. About 30 percent were infected through heterosexual contact with an HIV-positive partner. (In contrast, heterosexual contact was the means of transmission for only 2 percent of reported cases of men with AIDS.) Transfusion or treatment with contaminated blood products was responsible for about 10 percent of the cases.

Currently, AIDS is the largest cause of death for women between the ages of 25 and 34 in New York City. According to an epidemiological study in the April 17, 1987 issue of the *Journal of the American Medical Association*, New Jersey and Florida have the second and third largest number of women with AIDS, followed by California. The states with the highest proportion of women with AIDS, in terms of total AIDS cases, are New Jersey and Connecticut (each 16 percent), Puerto Rico (12 percent), Florida and Rhode Island (11 percent) and New York (10 percent).

Canada has reported 1,775 cases. Eighty percent of the Canadian cases are among gay/bisexual men. Only 3 percent of the cases are linked to IV drug use, compared to 22 percent in the United States.

Africa

The transmission patterns in Africa have differed from those of the northern hemisphere since the beginning of the pandemic. In Africa, AIDS is as prevalent among women as men, and some countries have reported more cases of women with AIDS than men. Blood transfusions and heterosexual contact with an infected partner are believed to be the main modes of transmission. All kinds of other explanations have been given, from promiscuity to female circumcision, from imperialistic genocidal intentions to the use of unclean needles. These explanations have neither provided a satisfactory answer nor prompted a concerted international effort to prevent the spreading of the virus. As of October 1987, Uganda (2,369 cases) and Tanzania (1,608 cases) are the two African countries with the most reported cases, followed by Kenya and Congo. North Africa has the smallest number of AIDS cases in the region.

Caribbean

The Caribbean is one of the most seriously affected regions in the world. In March 1988, Haiti headed the list with 1,374 cases, followed by 504 in the Dominican Republic. In these two countries transmission seems to be mostly heterosexual, while Trinidad's 227 cases were mostly among gay/bisexual men. In Bermuda the 75 reported cases are mostly composed of IV drug users.

Latin America

The Latin American country with the highest reported numbers of cases is Brazil with 2,956 cases, followed by Mexico with 1,302 cases. In both countries gay/bisexual men make up most of the cases. Contaminated blood and blood products have helped to spread the virus into the general population.

Pacific

Australia heads the statistics from this region with 813 cases, followed by New Zealand with 77 cases. Most of these cases are found among gay men, some are due to contaminated blood, and less than 1 percent to drug use.

Asia

Only 21 Asian countries had reported AIDS cases to WHO by March 1988. Of these, Japan (66 cases), Israel (58 cases), Qatar (32 cases), and Turkey (21 cases) were among the highest. Apart from Israel, where both contaminated blood and homosexual contact were the categorized modes of transmission, all the other countries indicated that it was mostly contaminated blood that caused infection. The cases of homosexual transmission were among foreigners or people who had lived abroad.

Europe

In the spring of 1988, Albania was the only European country without a single reported AIDS case. France heads the European statistics with 3,628 cases, making it the second-ranking internationally. West Germany has reported 1,973 cases, Italy 1,865 cases, and Britain 1,429 cases. Initially the virus was spread through homosexual contact, but during the last couple of years infection among IV drug users has risen sharply, accounting for more than half of the cases in Italy and Spain. Although the number of cases is lower in Switzerland, Belgium, and Denmark, all have reported between 263 to 439 cases, the rates of per capita infection in those countries, along with France, are the highest in Europe. Throughout Eastern Europe few AIDS cases have been reported — 4 in the Soviet Union, 3 in Poland, and 12 in Hungary — and they were mostly attributed to foreigners who, according to government officials, were quickly sent back home.

These realities and facts describe only one aspect of the AIDS story. The accounts presented in this anthology demonstrate the real impact of this epidemic on our lives.

I

Family, Lovers and Friends

IN TIMES OF crisis — and disease is a crisis — we need people to fall back on. Depending on the circumstances, we choose our biological families, our lovers, or our friends to be with us and help us. Since an AIDS diagnosis carries a stigma, families of people with AIDS are forced to confront many problems besides those of a life-threatening disease. In many cases, they have to deal with the sexual preference of the diagnosed person for the first time, or the fact that someone close to them has been using IV drugs.

Taking on the responsibility of physically caring for a relative, lover or close friend who has been diagnosed with AIDS often ends up being a woman's task. When making this commitment, though, few are prepared for what lies ahead of them. Their own lives often come to a standstill, revolving around someone else's needs twenty-four hours a day.

There are many people with AIDS who are left out in the cold, with no place to go. Either they are unable to talk to relatives or friends, or they simply don't have people to be with them when they are most in need. Support networks, often founded and staffed by people who have already dealt with a family member, lover or friend with AIDS, have stepped in and taken on their care — emotionally, financially and physically.

Not all the women writing in this chapter have taken care of a person with AIDS. But they all were affected — personally or politically — by a family member's or a friend's AIDS diagnosis. Each of them has had to confront issues of sexuality, society's reaction to the disease, or their own mortality.

Not in My House

R. MAYER

*The following account was written in the fall of 1987. R. Mayer, a
social work administrator in New York, describes the effects of her husband
Tom's AIDS diagnosis on her family.*

W E DRIVE TO see the snow, to
show Sam what snow looks and feels like. He's fallen asleep, so we keep
riding through back roads. The snow glistens, looks plump and puffy
on all it has touched.

"I think I have it," Tom says.

"Why," I ask, staring ahead. "What makes you think that?"

"There's a mark on my arm, it was a shadow but now it's become a
purplish mark. It's Kaposi's, I'm sure of it."

When Sam awakens, we stop at our favorite restaurant. It looks
down the river past the George Washington Bridge. The snow is
sparse here; we crunch to the water's edge, point to snow patches for
Sam to touch. No second child, I think.

That was December 1986.

I awaken from a dream. My father's hand reaches out through the
clouds and slaps me. "How could you have married someone like
that?" "I didn't marry 'someone like that,' I married a person who
loved me. I know he had a past, I knew that risk. I didn't know his past
had this kind of future."

Tom sits on the couch staring. He has no energy but watches Sam
play as though he were watching a movie. He says he is tired and can't
move but he's not sick.

One night we talk about the future. "It will be all right," he assures
me. "Everything will work out."

"No, no, it's not all right," I cry into his arms. For the first time we cry
together. Then we talk about his death. Who gets what, whom to call
first. He wants his ashes scattered. We don't talk about what will happen in between.

This is my disease, I think. This disease is a statement of life. I don't
have the virus but I have the disease. It's a disease of exposure. It's a
disease that tells people about Tom's past and therefore mine. I feel
tainted and ashamed.

I worry that Sammy could be sick. I call our doctor, then call the pediatric AIDS hotline, not once but daily for a week. They reassure me. "If you don't have it, your son doesn't." I repeat that over and over again. People ask me, "But how can you be so sure?" My aunt says, "It's hard to imagine that in our family. I'm so sorry to say that." Her daughter says, "What if Sammy bites my daughter?" And her sister says we can visit for an hour. Two of her three children are not at home. We sit stiffly in her chilly living room and make conversation.

We tell our families first. One by one. Though they are not surprised, they are shocked. At first they are supportive; later they will pull away. We tell certain friends. The ones with children. We fear Sam could be left out. But we are lucky; no one says we should stay at home.

Through January, Tom remains healthy. He goes to California to visit his father and sister. He wants their support and wants them to see him healthy. By late January, he has become more moody, withdrawn. The California trip has worn off. He has lost some more weight and has developed a terrible cough, which he says is post-nasal drip. He refuses to talk and refuses to call the doctor about the cough.

The smell of herbal cough drops nauseates me. It clings to the air.

Sammy knows something is going on. He runs to his room and into his crib where he clutches his doll and monkey. He talks to them. I don't know what to tell him. At two and a half years old, what will he understand?

Tom becomes obsessed with eating the right food. There is no treatment for Kaposi's sarcoma and he feels time is slipping away. He grouses about the empty refrigerator. I start to cook. No matter what I make, he says it's not what he has a taste for, it's not what he wants.

During the night, he has cold sweats, the other reminder of illness. The smell coats the bedroom. One night, he wakes up, soaked. He wants my help, but I am furious with him. I am angry that he is weak, angry that I don't sleep through the night any more. He coughs and rattles the bed and I wake up. Sammy calls for me. Many nights I fall asleep exhausted on the couch at 5:00 a.m.

"What if he dies; how will I manage?" I think. After Tom and Sammy fall asleep, I wander through our house and one night go into Tom's office. I look for information — names of insurance companies, account numbers, anything that will tell me about our finances. I berate myself because these are the things that he manages, and if something happens to him I won't know what to do. I also fear living without a supporter; I fear being independent and raising our son alone. I worry that my salary isn't enough and so think about working two jobs.

"Tom," I ask one night, "tell me where things are. Who handles the insurance, who is our insurance agent. I need the bank account numbers."

"Not now. I can't do that. It's all in the file cabinet, just look for it."

"No. I want to go over it with you. I need your help with this."

"I have to go back to work. Later. It's not important now. I'm still here. I don't know what's so important. It's all here. Stop worrying, you're always worrying about something."

I remember the look on my mother's face after my father died. It was sudden; no one was prepared, least of all my mother. Papers were strewn on the dining room table for weeks. Bills piled up. I watched her put her life together by going through those papers. That myriad of detailed information that she never dealt with. She looked confused, then determined. I felt that by asking I was intruding, making something out of nothing.

Some nights, I need to get out, to be with friends. When I leave, Tom coughs louder, sputters and looks pained. "Drink tea," I yell, "take cough medicine." I walk out the door as fast as I can.

On the phone, he tells people he's doing fine, working hard. He talks about research studies that he's investigating, tells them he thinks there are going to be things out there for him. He reads constantly now, listens for every scrap of information and tells his doctor his theories. His doctor is impressed with his knowledge.

Off the phone, he is silent, picky. One night I yell at him, "Get out of here, go some place." He yells back, "No, you go."

"I've been gone all day, you leave." I storm around him; he puts on the television earphones and lies on the couch with arms crossed.

Something else has to happen. I am constantly angry now; I can't stand his helplessness. I can't give him sympathy or companionship any more. Something else has to happen.

I dream about a woman who has three children with AIDS. She runs from one to the other, touching them, feeding them, making them comfortable. She is confused, tired.

Sammy and I are sitting at the table. It is Friday night, the Sabbath. We sit looking at the glowing candles, the flowers. He says, "I'm sad."

"Why are you sad, Sammy?"

"Because Mommy's sad."

I sit up straight. "Sometimes Mommy feels sad." I pause. "You know that Daddy has not been feeling well."

He laughs and fidgets. "He's been coughing a lot lately. You've heard him cough. It bothers him now." He looks at me and makes a funny face, dances in his seat, then gets down and runs to his room. "Run, Mommy, run."

Saturday night. It's March now. Tom sits hunched in the corner of the couch. Our friends are over. The house is lively. Sammy goes up to them, "You come to my room?" Tom looks pained. I sit with him and put my arm around his thin shoulders. He clutches me. His breathing is so labored he can barely get from one end of the house to the other. He has finally called the doctor, who says to wait until some test results come back; right now there is nothing definitive. Nothing except his growing inability to walk more than a few steps at a time; then he has to stop and gasp for air. He says it will go away.

The doctor says it's pneumonia. Tom insists on staying home to take the medicine, which makes him sick. He stays in bed for the weekend. Monday morning, he throws up, but tells me he will be all right. I go to work, walk in, walk out, go home and call the doctor to get him into the hospital. I remember later that Sammy had seen all of this. He saw his Daddy barely able to move out of bed, saw him throw up, saw us take his Daddy to the hospital while my sister stayed with him. Sammy insisted on watching it all. While we waited for the doctor to call back, he said, "When I get big can I have cough drops?"

"Maybe you'll want other food, like quiche or escargot."

"Yeah," he nods, "I can have quiche, and cough drops."

No Patience to Go On Complaining

MARGARETH

Marlene Rodrigues interviewed Margareth, a film producer, in January 1988, in São Paulo, Brazil.

IN OUR FAMILY we are four brothers and sisters. Roberto was the oldest, and he was the one closest to me. I learned a lot from him; he taught me to listen to music, and from age ten he gave me Russian and French novels to read. He was a very tender person, very interesting, very beautiful.

When he turned twenty, he left our city in the Northeast and came to São Paulo to work and study. He lived at the YMCA, and it was there that he met a young American who had come to Brazil on a Rotary Club cultural exchange program. They became very close, and in 1968 Roberto left for the United States. He enrolled in the University of Texas, studied languages and American literature, and worked as a cook in a restaurant. Roberto liked health food and was a very good cook.

My mother died in 1973, while Roberto was living in New York. When I finally managed to track him down to tell him of her death, she was already buried. He was desperate — he was the first-born and very close to her. He decided to pack up and come back. While he was getting ready to move back, our father became sick and he, too, died before Roberto's arrival. These losses were too much, and I don't think he ever recuperated from them.

Roberto returned to Brazil, and for a year he lived with me and my children in Salvador. By that time I had split up with my husband. Living with Roberto did not work out well, because he always interfered with the raising of my kids. He wanted to bring them up like little Americans, and I couldn't stand it. I've always had problems with American culture — I still do. I don't know if it is because of the kind of life my brother led, or if it is because I associate his getting this disease with his life in America. I just know that I despise that hot dog culture. After leaving Salvador, he went to São Paulo and started working as a technical translator. I always thought of him as a healthy person, practicing karate, jogging, and eating vegetarian food.

He had come out in the United States. He was a pretty difficult person — he had his private life locked away in his house, in his own world. I talked with him about it when he returned to Brazil. He had come back alone. He was never committed to a relationship; he was always promiscuous. He had never lived with anyone; he was pretty complicated in those matters, always thinking that his partners tried to take advantage of him. He was a loner, and I think all his relationships remained very superficial.

I perceived all this much later when I started to take care of him, even though I had already sensed that his way of dealing with people was very different from mine. I think life goes on showing us things which we filter and incorporate. Within Roberto there was an emotional split which made me worry. Of course, people behave in different ways depending on where they are — at work, in bars, or at home, but these are just nuances. Every time he came for a visit, and I invited him to go to the theater, the movies or a show, he would decline. He was only interested in slipping out of his body, his clothes, the armor of his work as a technical translator, and to put on the cloak of promiscuity.

He would come home at dawn, and I had no idea where he had been. I thought of him as my oldest son, rather than my brother. Deep down I thought that something bad would happen to him. I never thought that he would get sick, but I thought of something like a murder, that he would be killed one day by someone whom he picked up.

In 1984, Roberto started complaining about memory loss and severe headaches. That year he went to New York for a vacation and he fell sick there. A big tumor was discovered in the left side of his brain, and he had to be taken home. He was admitted to a private clinic in São Paulo. The doctors asked for a copy of the medical records from the United States, and Roberto, in a panic, said, "I had all the tests done, even the one for AIDS, and I don't think it's anything serious." But since he hadn't brought back any of the records, and since the doctors were alerted, they tested him, and the result was positive. Then the situation became very complicated. Since he had the virus, they isolated him from all the other patients. In order to enter his room, everyone was required to wear a mask and special clothes.

They operated on him and removed the tumor. Roberto was very strong physically, and since he hadn't shown any signs of AIDS-related symptoms, he recuperated quickly and underwent radiation treatments. But from then on, and maybe because of the radiation, he began having problems which had nothing to do with the operation. He had fevers which would come and go and extreme sweats which left his bed soaking wet and smelling really foul, a smell of death. Even remembering it makes me sick.

After the operation and the radiation, Roberto went back to work. But after about six months, he quit his job. When the doctors did further testing, they discovered a new tumor, bigger than the first one. The doctors told me that they wouldn't operate again, because there was no point to it. Roberto had AIDS symptoms, and was getting worse day by day.

I had the impression that Roberto really didn't want to know about the reality of his situation, and we had to respect his wishes. Sometimes he would pressure me, wanting to know if he had something serious, and I would say, "I think so, but we are still not sure. Let's wait for the results of the next test." We can't just leave others with the impression that all will be right, or that all will be bad; we have to find some middle ground so that the sick can keep up hope. Otherwise, it becomes too overwhelming and exhausting.

Up until the first signs of Kaposi's sarcoma, his mind was still in good shape, and I made it clear to him what that sarcoma was all about. He just focused on that cancer, and refused to think any more about AIDS. I think that was wise; it was the glorious excuse to turn away from AIDS — the bogeyman, the true ghost of his life.

I took care of Roberto. I was the only one around to do it. He had friends, but the majority were superficial relations, people who were not in a position to fight shoulder to shoulder with him. From time to time, when I could leave him for a couple of hours, I went to bars, drank, listened to music, talked to people. This was my way of recharging. It was much more difficult for him, because his gay friends had a hard time dealing with the situation. For them it was like looking into a mirror and seeing their own reflection, wondering, "Will I end up like this?" I tried to spare them from doing things that would be too painful for them.

It all happened quite fast. Within a year he went from being a healthy person to living with death day in and day out. The tumor had debilitated him, and his identity was disintegrating. He was an educated person who spoke four or five languages, had been to Europe, had lived abroad for several years; the disease damaged what he considered to be his most important attributes: his lifestyle and his memory.

I had to develop a special way of communicating with him because his ability to speak had been destroyed. His reasoning was affected and so were his senses. In the end all that was left was "Eti," which was my childhood nickname. This was the name he called out when he was already in a coma.

When his health deteriorated even further, I tried to find a place in a hospital for him. Private hospitals don't have AIDS wards, and they didn't want to accept him. They suggested I send him to a public hospital with a ward for contagious and infectious diseases.

Roberto could not be left alone in his flat, so I brought him back to mine. But I had neither financial nor physical capabilities to take care of him. I had a back problem, due to the pressure I was under, and often I managed to move around only if I was holding on to furniture or the walls to help propel myself along.

Roberto stayed at my house for two days, and it was sheer madness. I had to put padlocks on all the doors and windows because he wanted to jump out. I live on the upper floor of an apartment building, but he thought he was on the ground floor. He had lost the notion of danger.

It is quite a responsibility to deal with a person who has lost his memory, who no longer knows what is going on. A woman who used to be my babysitter and who knew about Roberto's disease came to help me. I tried to find a number of nurses to care for him, but it didn't work out. The pressures on me increased, and I felt as if I were being buried by an avalanche. Those few days were the apex, the nuclear bomb exploding my limits.

He started to have diarrhea, couldn't take a bath on his own, and no longer knew when to go to the bathroom. He soiled his pants and the bed, and I had to struggle with him. I even had to hit him, take off his clothes, and force him to take a bath. Roberto was enormous; he hadn't lost any weight, and weighed about 180 pounds. Sometimes he tried to attack me, giving me karate blows. In the end I couldn't stand it anymore, and I decided to put him back into the hospital. This hadn't been my intention; I had tried to find a way so that he could stay at home. But this would have cost me a fortune, money I didn't have. And, on top of it, I just didn't have the physical ability to keep someone in my flat who was practically in a coma.

Two of his women friends contacted the administration of the Emilio Ribas Hospital (São Paulo's largest public hospital, the only one with an AIDS ward), and I found a place for him there. That was a feat, because there are many sick people and very few beds. The trip in the ambulance from my house to the hospital was my last ride with my brother through the city of São Paulo.

And then another problem arose. Two days after Roberto was hospitalized, I was called in for an interview with the doctor in charge. This doctor didn't receive me in his office, but at the hospital's entrance. And right there, among all these people, he showed me a paper saying that my brother couldn't stay longer: "Your brother has terminal cancer — he can't stay here."

"But my brother has AIDS."

"He's only in the beginning stages of AIDS. We need to keep these beds for people who are in a much more advanced stage of the disease."

"Do you know anything about my life? Do you know that my brother is single, and that there is nobody to take care of him, and he is practically in a coma? Do you know that he always paid his taxes, and that his social security and health insurance were taken out of his salary his entire life? You are not going to kick him out of here. If you do this, I will make a big scene right here in the hospital."

We had a long discussion, but when he saw that I was really mad, he got scared and sent me to talk with a social worker. I negotiated with her and got a week's grace period in order to set up everything to take care of Roberto at home again. From then on, every time I arrived at the hospital, the functionaries would ask me when I was going to take him home. The pressure was so strong that I hoped he would get worse and die soon. I was forced to think contrary to my emotions as a sister. This was one of the worst things ever to happen to me. Every time Roberto would get better, the story of taking him home was brought up again. It went on for two months, and then he died.

Shortly after Roberto's death in 1986, I had myself tested for AIDS, even though my doctor said that it wasn't necessary. It took lots of courage to open up the envelope with the result, but luckily it was negative. This made me feel that I had returned to life, and from then on, I began to pick up the joy of life again.

Our passage through life is very temporary, and we need to gain as much as we can from it. Sometimes good things happen, and then there are other moments which are difficult, and we have to confront them. I don't have any patience to go on complaining. I believe in life and the emotions of life. I don't think of myself as a superwoman, but after the experience I've gone through, I've developed a sense of my own strength.

Mine was one of those typical marriages to please my family. Still, I had such a strong sense of freedom! I was one of those wild girls who went swimming, fishing and running. My sense of freedom comes from the child within me, and because she is free, without rules, she has her own discipline for life.

In the seventies, after my parents' deaths, my marriage fizzled out. I felt as if the production of a film had come to its end, and I, the leading actress, said, "I'm sorry, but my contract is over; let's get back to reality." Leaving my marriage paved the way to a new world, professionally as well as sexually. I was in therapy, and I ended up involved with my analyst, who was a woman. This caused such a scandal in my town!

Sometimes I sit here thinking, reviewing the old "films" of my life. I see myself as a special person, not out of vanity, but because I have the courage to confront the world. When I had to deal with the crisis of losing my brother, I had already met other crises. Taking care of Roberto, I seized the unknown, the phantom that was there, inside of him. There are moments in life when it is impossible to go into reverse gear.

But more important than the fear of the disease itself — and I was afraid — was dealing with the fact that I had always been my brother's only source of support. In my relationship with him, I restrained my own femininity on some level, in order for his to come out. Our relationship was so strong, and he wanted to be me. I think he really wanted to be a woman, but I didn't want to be a man. I've always enjoyed being a woman: I am strong, quarrelsome. I don't like to hide problems, but prefer to confront them, and at the same time I like to play out my tender side, my femininity. Roberto and I had had defined roles ever since our childhood: since I am the stronger one, I had to stand firm, waiting to support him from behind the scenes, while he was acting on stage.

Throughout his illness, these things came up again, and they were more sharply defined than ever. I had to make all the decisions, and he behaved like a spoiled girl. He made me buy some knickknacks for him to play with, and he talked to them, putting them on the window sill and on the furniture. He spent hours arranging a set of white china on the shelves, and he forbade me to touch it, as if I was a father who didn't understand its delicacy. I respected his behavior because we should have respect for those who are leaving. He was searching for the stereotypical model of the female soul, a farfetched, rococo image of woman.

I think that my brother's death allowed me to distance myself from my role in our relationship. Suddenly I could be myself, and my emotional needs changed. Before I was very speedy, I wanted everything immediately, but today I'm quite different. I think things over for a while before I get involved. I don't want to be in a relationship for social reasons, or out of fear of being alone, or out of habit. I have reorganized my priorities. I am no longer content with a relationship that is simply sexual; I want to be entirely involved. Then I feel complete.

Lately, I've also realized how much I've lived my life for other people over the past twenty years. Professionally, for example, I'm working in a field in which, in terms of my age, I am twenty years behind most of my peers. I had a husband, I raised my kids, I made and lost money. I left my life in Rio de Janeiro in order to come and take care of my brother. Now that I am reaching forty, I can finally be myself.

I'm still exhausted after all this. Often I think that I'm in the hospital with Roberto. I was so removed from the world, and even today I have a hard time being interested in what is happening around me. I have made sure that I don't hear anything about AIDS. I have had such a horrible experience with this disease, with the hospitals, with the doctors, with the prejudice; everything was so bad that I don't have the slightest desire to talk to anyone about it. I'm tired of it.

Dying With Dignity

JUDI STONE

Judi Stone was born in Rumania to Hungarian parents and raised in Venezuela. Her son, Michael, was diagnosed with AIDS in September 1984. He died only two months later, at the age of nineteen. Soon after Michael's death, Judi quit her job at a museum, and began work on a social welfare degree. She is AIDS Volunteer Coordinator at San Francisco's Kaiser Hospital and an emotional support counselor and group leader for the Shanti Project. Ines Rieder spoke with her on January 19, 1988.

IT WAS 1984, AND I hadn't yet heard of people my son's age dying of AIDS. I thought that he was too young and strong, and that he would live through it. Teenagers deal with death so much better than those of us who are older. Michael said, "I am not depressed, I am not giving up, but it is a fact that I will die. So what did you bring me for lunch?" Everything was very matter-of-fact. He faced the issue of dying — but what could he do about it?

At the beginning of November, the month he died, Michael asked me to do his Christmas shopping. He gave me a list of things to buy. I wanted to know why he wanted to do it then. And he said, "Mother, you know that I won't be around; why don't you just listen?"

Teenagers don't realize the finality of death. They haven't lived long enough to know what they will have lost. For them, being thirty is old age. What they are losing is not something they are looking forward to. It's much easier for them.

My husband had a real hard time. He didn't have any hope. He realized right at the beginning that Michael was going to die. For the first few weeks he took to drinking. Every night he would drink to put himself to sleep. He was out like a light by 8:30. He became very withdrawn. I was talking and going to support groups. At that time I worked at the Fine Arts Museum, and I was working with people. He had an office by himself and he didn't have to talk to anyone. I realized what was going on, and I thought that he needed to spend time with Michael.

Michael got along with his father, but they didn't talk very much. I had a long talk with Ralph, my husband, and I said, "You have two choices: either you stop drinking, and you start spending more time with Michael, or you can move out. I don't want you in the house if you go on like this." Mind you, we had been married for over twenty-four years and it's a happy marriage. That was a hard choice. And he hasn't had a drink since. He ended up spending more time with Michael than I did.

When Michael was in the hospital, I used to call him every morning, until he said, "Mother don't call me in the morning." I stopped. Now that I've been around the hospital so long, I realize that people often don't get to sleep until 3:00 or 4:00 in the morning, and calling them at 8:00 means waking them up. I never felt that it was a personal offense when he said, "Mother, I'm tired. Would you go home?" And if I come to think of it, if I was sick and dying, I wouldn't want my mother there twenty-four hours a day. I don't think I would want my husband there twenty-four hours a day.

Michael didn't want anyone to know that he had AIDS. I think something traumatized him in that hospital in Santa Cruz. Was it because of all the masks and gowns, or was it some religious person who came and spoke to him? They had said that someone should come in and give him the last rites. We told them that he wasn't religious, and that it wouldn't be appropriate. When we transferred him to San Francisco's Kaiser Hospital, he asked me, "Mother, would you make sure that no religious nut comes to bother me?"

Michael had had a relationship with a man for four or five years and he wouldn't allow me to tell him about his illness. Peter would call here and want to know about Michael. I wasn't allowed to tell him that Michael was sick and in the hospital. And Michael forbade us to tell our families.

He finally told his best friend, Albert, who was very loving and caring. And little by little he would tell other people. But when they called, he would say, "I can't talk now, I'll call back." And then he never called back. And when people came for visits, he would say, "I have no time now. Could you please go?" He spent lots of time with Sheera, his Shanti buddy, but only while he was at home. And he never called his friend Peter. After Michael's death, I called Peter and told him what had happened.

When Michael died, we told his grandmother that he had died of Hodgkin's disease. Later we told her the truth, and I was glad that the truth was out, though she never talks about him.

My relatives can't deal with homosexuality. As a matter of fact, my father and my brother still don't know that Michael died of AIDS. I never told them. When I had told my mother that Michael was sick, she just drove me crazy: "How did you let him get sick?" It was as if it was my fault.

My family lives in West Germany now, and I didn't think that there was any need to say more. My father and my brother were here for a visit last summer, and if they had asked me, I would have told them. And Ralph's family, in the South, reacted in a way that made us think it would have been better not to have said anything.

We had been on television, and then there was an interview with us in the Shanti newsletter. They were going to find out, and it was better that they found out through us. By the time we told Ralph's brother, he already knew, since someone had told him we'd been on television talking about Michael's death. But they don't talk about it. What was the hardest for them to accept was the fact that there was no funeral. Michael was cremated and his ashes are in the back yard. I asked Michael what he wanted me to do with his ashes, and he said, "Mother, you be creative, do whatever you want to do." I used them as a fertilizer, and I planted three bottlebrushes. I believe in recycling; life goes on in different forms.

Michael died on the Sunday after Thanksgiving. Then at Christmas time, when the relatives knew how hard it was, you would think that they would have called. I have to be fair with them; it's not just dealing with AIDS, they have problems dealing with death. People have problems talking about it. And they don't realize that this makes it even worse.

I believe that a person only really dies when we forget him; when we never talk about him, it's as if he never existed. We are all going to die, and we might as well accept it. I talk to Michael sometimes. Maybe I don't talk out loud, but in my mind I do.

Losing a child is different from losing a parent, a husband or a brother. You always expect that you'll lose your parents, because they are older. But your children are supposed to outlive you. And by losing them, you lose part of yourself.

I took it real hard after he died — I came down with pneumonia myself. Stress can really do you in. For four months I went to my Shanti group meeting, and I did a lot of physical things. I refinished the floors and stripped the staircase. I went back to work at the museum, but after being back for three days, I decided that I couldn't handle it, and that's when I took a year's leave of absence.

Since I am a photographer, Shanti asked me to do some photography for them. Then I became involved in their speakers group. They needed me since I was a parent — there are not that many parents out in the open.

I volunteered to put together educational material about AIDS. And then I met someone who had just been coming in on his own to visit AIDS patients at Kaiser Hospital, where Michael had died. I thought it might be good to have a support program. After having started a group, I also became an emotional support volunteer at with Shanti. Then I facilitated trainings for a group called The Most Holy Redeemer, which is like Shanti, but smaller. I also got involved with the public school system to promote AIDS education. I've testified before both the Human Rights Commission and the school board. After having done all this, my year was up, and I decided that I didn't really want to go back to the museum. I was more interested in working with terminally ill people.

I now coordinate a group of nineteen volunteers at Kaiser Hospital. Most of them have been there for a year or more. The volunteers come to the hospital at least three hours a week, and participate in a monthly support group meeting.

If a patient asks the family to come, they come, at least in the majority of the cases. Keep in mind that most patients at Kaiser's are gay. We have had only one woman so far, and one baby. Kaiser has been good to its AIDS patients. I haven't heard of any attempts to cancel people from the plan after they have been diagnosed.

I've seen many fights between lovers and families. The families often blame the lovers: *if it wasn't for you, my son wouldn't be gay.* I had one gay couple who had been together for thirty-four years, and then the family came in and didn't treat the lover as they would treat a spouse. In situations like this, we try to intervene and ask the family to back off. We ask the patient what he wants, and try to get the family to respect his decisions.

Usually I have Latino clients because I am bilingual. When Latino families deal with each other's illnesses and deaths, it's quite different. Even if they don't get along, they all come in, and they stick by the relative who is ill. They don't talk about the person being gay, but they are there.

If someone wants to hang on to life, to every little hope, I wholeheartedly support that. But what I get from patients who have had AIDS for a year, a couple of years, even six or seven months, and who are not doing well, is this: "I wish I could just let it go, and be over with it. But my lover thinks if I eat differently or if I take this medication I'll be O.K. My parents want me to hang on since there might be something around the corner; they want me to take AZT." Some of these people should be allowed to just let go.

I don't think any of us knows what it is like to live like that. Sometimes lying around in bed and going to the bathroom takes all your effort and eats up all your energy for the day. And when you get to the point when you can't even do that, and somebody has to do it for you, all you do is lie there. You are in pain, or you are not totally clear, because your pain medications make you a bit confused. You are just there, vegetating. That's not quality of life.

I have a very strong personal belief in people's right to die with dignity. I don't believe in being heroic. I don't believe that the longer you live the better it is. I believe in quality, even if it's for a short time period. Michael died in the way that was good for him. A couple hours before he died, he went to the bathroom by himself, and he was still talking to us, which is totally different from the people who are kept alive on machines. His words were: "I want to get something massive and get it over with. I don't want to stay in bed for months." He didn't want to go on a respirator. He preferred to die with dignity.

About Going Home

DYANA BASIST

For John Walsh, who died September 24, 1987 of AIDS.

I.

I'd been puttin it off for five days, been busy with life, things, makin
plans. So this morning I called John in some hospital in
New York city and there was something in his voice;
seemed thin and desert dry.
I said, "Hey Walsh, this is Big." Big's what he calls me: Big Dy.
I knew him before I changed my name and he vowed to call me
Diane forever. We finally settled on Big. I like the name cause
I feel big. People keep telling me I'm skinny, fragile. One guy
even thought I was anorexic. Inside me, I'm big, real big and full.

John told me, "You know I've been shittin for weeks, can't keep
anything down. I snuck some Welch's grape juice, it's my favorite,
puked my guts out for four hours. Christ, I just had a little sip.
I got all these visitors — piling in, god, ya just never
know ya have so many friends.
They did another biopsy and found cancer in my stomach."
His voice became wind — could hardly hear him.
He started crying. "You know, I have to decide if I should
get this operation. I'm weak, those other operations made me
real tired. The doctors, god, oh Big, there's this pain.
I gotta go. I can't talk." I tell him I'll call him tomorrow.
"Yeah, Big, tomorrow."

Walked six miles on the beach yesterday. It was windy but I
went in anyway and it felt great. Always does — cold and salty,
all that salt.
Today, I collected food from the garden and made things. My mother
told me, "When you feel bad just keep cooking." She made three
pots of soup when her mother died last year. Had to give a lot of it
away. Three pots in four days. Today I made gazpacho,
three-bean salad, pear sauce and peach crisp.

36

II.

I wake up. It's dark. Acorns fall on the corrugated plastic roof.
Roosters crow. Turn in bed — over and over, hands under chin,
hands warm between thighs. Still never know what to do with my
moving hands. I know if I could just quiet these fingers,
the rest would follow.
I think of John in Roosevelt Hospital, maybe he's keepin me
awake. I talk myself past John, until the night traffic
becomes the shush of ocean waves and then no sound, save my
expected breath.
I don't want to call him today, but I do. I say, "John, it's Big."
"This isn't John."
"Yes it is," I argue.
The voice sounds almost the same; like vines holding onto
buildings. Ivy covering windows. I call back to the same reply.
After innumerable phone calls, I reach his nurse in intensive care.
He's alive, she isn't supposed to tell me, but god I'm calling
from California. He's stable, very weak. She'll tell him I called.

I can see the garden. The sunflowers which took on the second
planting are strong-stemmed, taller than me, about to open
yellow, heavy, and bend under their own weight.
In the kitchen, the white rose I stuck in water a week ago
continues to drop petals, big and soft as my cheek, onto
the counter and red tiled floor.

III.

There's a message on my answering machine
that he's dead

                        information I take down a number
feel nothing

I lay down   wait to feel something
and wait

               get up   take a shower
go to sleep

up at 4 a.m.
lay there
nothing   my body is long and sharp
nothing.

He died when I was backpacking. I was calm that day.
Had driven 7 hours, hiked 12 miles with 30 lbs
just to get that still.
I lay on a rock. The aspens were turning gold, orange.
I thought about having a child. Saw a hawk, deer, bear tracks.
Bathed in hot springs until rain pushed me under cedars.
Never thought about him all day. Not once.

Before I left, I called, he said: "I'm going home next Thursday.
They're taking me by ambulance cause I can't sit up. My fever's down
to 101, after two weeks it just went down."

His voice was shaking like those aspens brilliant

He knew he was dying   spinning tight with fear
              snap   falling scattered on
the forest floor

the night he was going home   going home

They say you die like you live. He told me, "I'm gonna fight
my brains out. Be one of the lucky ones."

In the garden, the beans have shriveled brown up the bamboo.
Tomatoes rot into the earth, peppers mold. I want everything dead,
but incessantly these wildflowers bloom.

again
up at 4:00 a.m.

all sounds are sudden
everything is happening for the first time
nothing is enough.

Ten Thousand Waves

PAZ

I FEEL THE PAIN and grief all through my husband's illness and the memories after his death come and wash over me, not like a tidal wave but as ten thousand waves, one after the other — never seeming to cease.

Larry, my husband of twenty years, died on August 10, 1987 after a sixteen-month battle with AIDS. My children and I greatly miss him and we are slowly realizing how much our lives have been affected by his death.

We were very fortunate because people responded to his disease with love and concern, and helped make his passing from life to death the best it could have been. To comprehend this, one has to understand the phenomenon of death as a pulling away of the soul from the body, and the dying process as a letting go of so many parts of one's individual identity — item by item is put down and not addressed again as death nears. I watched and cared for him and saw a strong and active, forty-year-old man's body and mind deteriorate to a point where he needed assistance with nearly everything. The last three months of his life were spent with little strength and little clarity.

I had met Larry in 1966 in Eugene, Oregon, where we both were trained as VISTA volunteers. We worked with Mexican-American migrant workers, helping them to find permanent jobs and homes. This was our first experience in working to counter social injustices, and Larry's life work was always related to improving the social conditions of others.

His career in health care allowed us to live and work in many different parts of the United States and three Latin American countries. In each of these countries one of our children was born. Our married life was full and active. Larry differed from most men because he was very gentle, and he deeply cared for our children. Although being married to him certainly did present challenges, required tolerance and at times caused me much pain, I have always loved him dearly and will never regret our marriage.

In January 1986, Larry returned from a business trip and announced that he wanted a divorce. At this point in our marriage we had been growing apart, but we certainly had withstood many crises — including his need for sex and love with men. All during February, he and I played the game of separating — I recall a few discussions of who would get what and who would care for whom. But nothing was ever settled. Now I think that he knew that he had been infected, and he wanted to spare me and our children the pain and ordeal of caring for him while dying. In March, he lost twenty-five pounds, developed a deep cough and was extremely fatigued. He went to see a doctor but did not tell him that he was at high risk for contracting AIDS.

I remember still being in the divorce frame of mind but knowing that something was very wrong. At the same time, he became frightened and wanted my company and comfort. One evening we were sitting together and he proceeded to tell me of all the medical tests that were being performed to find the cause of his mysterious weight loss and fatigue. His illness then was mysterious only because the doctors didn't know what to look for. I asked him if he had told his doctors that he belonged to one of the high-risk groups for AIDS. He hadn't, but the next day he found the courage to tell them. Immediately, a gallium scan was performed and a spot was found on his lung. He was hospitalized for a biopsy as well as treatment.

Larry tried hard to maintain a normal work schedule, and one day before entering the hospital, he finished building a trellis on our front porch. This was his last building project, and also his way of denying that he had AIDS.

What still amazes me is how he was able to deny his gayness, even to himself, and that he never acknowledged his relationships with men. The three men with whom he had long-term relationships were wonderful sources of strength for Larry and me during his illness. They are still good friends of mine, and I am sure that I'll always stay in contact with them.

Years ago, I accused Larry of using me and the children to cover his gayness. Even at that time, I knew that the accusation was unfair, and during the course of his illness and since his death, I have realized that the children and I were the center of his life. Although I needed more love, it was impossible for me to accept what love he did bring to our relationship. I was also unable to fully appreciate what I had, because I viewed our relationship in terms of a conventional marriage — which it was not.

In April 1986, Larry returned home from the hospital and tried to pick up the pieces of his life, which now had a huge cloud over every aspect of it. Many tears were shed by both of us and much time was spent reshaping what future we still had. At this point, a role reversal took place in our relationship. I took on more responsibility in terms of decision-making, and Larry became the more emotional and needing partner.

Those first months after his first stay in the hospital were very difficult. Larry did not want our friends to know what was wrong with him. He did, however, tell our two teenage sons (but not our youngest), and by telling them about his illness, he had to tell them of his past relationships with men. This was painful for all three, but it set the tone for a very open, caring relationship.

Larry continued working but was often very ill and unable to participate in normal family activities. His goal was to work through January 1987 so he could increase his employment-provided life insurance. But putting all energy into work left little energy for any other activities.

When AZT became available to the general public in November 1986, Larry began taking it. It made him extremely nauseous, and he developed dangerously high fevers, which were accompanied by debilitating chills and sweats. He was hospitalized to control the fevers and after two more modified attempts, it became clear that he would never be able to tolerate it. The doctors were rather puzzled by what seemed then like a unique reaction to the drug. We realized that he wouldn't be one of the lucky ones to benefit from AZT. This was very painful, but the experience of the fevers, chills, and nausea made me think that anything had to be better than the physical condition created by the drug, even if it meant we were giving up all hope for intervention.

Larry was able to work through February 1987. At that time, he was taking steroids, which masked some of the symptoms. His energy level was better for a while, but he remained depressed, and it was becoming increasingly evident that the disease was affecting his memory and his thinking abilities.

A close friend once said that the three aspects of Larry's personality which stood out most were his compassion for others, his wonderful sense of humor and his sharp mind. The disease had changed all that. His depression and the reality of the disease had dampened his sense of humor and now the disease was also taking away his keen mind. For me, this was the cruelest aspect of what the disease did to the man I had spent half of my life with. It was difficult to watch his physical deterioration, but to see my husband turn into a person who often would get lost on the way to the bathroom in our own home was heartbreaking.

By June, when I finished the school year, Larry had deteriorated to the point where he needed full-time care. I know in my heart that he had held onto whatever reserve of strength he had until I would be able to be home with him all of the time. It was at this point that I had to take over the monitoring of his food and medication. He also became increasingly resistant to leaving the house and sometimes even our bedroom. His world was closing in on him and he began to hear voices and have imaginary visitors. At that point, many of his professional friends received phone calls from him, and they would have long conversations about health care. Larry would be able to hold his own during the conversation until he would make a reference to the purple elephant in the closet. A rumor that Larry had suffered a nervous breakdown began to circulate. When I heard about it, I decided it was necessary to tell people that he had AIDS, that he wouldn't live much longer, and that the disease was affecting his mind.

Early on in the illness, Larry had asked me not to tell people what was wrong with him. He was still afraid of being rejected and exposed. But by then I felt there was no longer any point in keeping his secret. As I began telling people what he had, each and every one responded with loving support.

Larry was fortunate not to experience any of the rejections so often heard about with people with AIDS. I think that was due to the kind of relationships he had developed with his friends, and with his women friends especially, because he did not view them as possible conquests, but rather as equals. I was never jealous of any of the women friends he had over the years, because early on I understood how he related to them and why the women always cherished his friendship.

His very gentle nature remained intact right to his death. He had always avoided conflict and in some ways this had hindered our relationship, because all too often he would equate an expression of strong emotion with conflict and run away from the exchange. But his soul's gentleness made the daily physical care much easier than it would have been if he had been a different type of person. He felt such sorrow in having to be cared for so totally.

Larry often got up at night and wandered around the house. I would have to be near him or he might injure himself or go outside and get lost. Our friends and relatives, who came from New York, Colorado, and Michigan to help with his care, relieved me during the day so I could attend to our children and our other affairs.

However, in August it seemed necessary to hire a part-time attendant. This wasn't my idea as much as others' — who were more aware that Larry was deteriorating to a point where he needed to be lifted out of bed, needed to be bathed, and where his bedding needed to be changed often. I agreed and we hired a wonderful attendant who has cared for AIDS patients since 1982. Once the attendant was brought in, Larry sensed my exhaustion and the toll this ordeal was taking on all of us.

The night before Larry went into coma, a very close friend, a physician, came by and tried to convince me that Larry needed to be put into the hospital — that we were doing a great job of caring for him, but that neither I nor the children could go on much longer. This was the first time I considered hospitalizing him. I know he must have been aware of it, and this enabled him to let go, because the next morning, when I tried to wake him, he was comatose.

I called the family, and they all came immediately — to be with him during his final five days. For twenty-four hours a day he had companionship — we took turns rubbing and bathing him, talking to and sitting quietly with him, trying in every way to make his letting go of this life as loving and peaceful as possible. I thanked one of my friends who came at 2:00 a.m. to sit with him until 5:00 a.m. on two nights, and she summed up best how everyone felt by telling me that it was an honor to participate.

During his last days, Larry was unable to move or communicate. His eyes remained opened for the full five days. On three occasions he cried with me, and I know those tears were tears of love. He cried for the first time early on in the coma when I was talking to him of my love for him and asking his forgiveness for having become short-tempered with him and his illness. He cried for the second time on the fourth day, when a dear friend and I played a tape of music which two friends had prepared to sing at the funeral. And the third and final time was five minutes before he took his last breath. I was alone with him, and I knew that it was a signal that the end was nearing. I called the family members into the room and we all held him as he passed from his life.

Soon after his death, people began to come to the house and pay their last respects. There was much sorrow, but also much love and a deep sense of relief that the long ordeal was over for Larry — all the pain from the illness, but also the pain of his life, keeping his secret and living a double life. A great weight was lifted from my shoulders when I was able to tell people the truth about what was killing him. By opening up about Larry, I was able to heal much of my hurt and confusion surrounding his gayness.

It has been three and a half months since my husband died. Our oldest son is very angry because his father left him. Our middle son is very depressed over having lost his father, and our eight-year-old daughter seems relieved from the stress the illness created in her. She was very close to him, and she is very lucky to have two older brothers who love her and who, I hope, will fill some of the great void created by her father's death.

Seeing him suffer was painful for me, but now I have to deal with the even greater pain of having lost the one I shared more than half my life with. I loved Larry greatly, and by having cared for him during his last months our love was affirmed. As time passes, I become more and more aware how tightly interwoven our lives were, and often I experience a great sense of confusion without his presence. Many well-meaning people tell me that as time passes it will get easier — perhaps it will — but I do know a very significant part of myself has died.

There is a cruel irony which creates much sorrow when I think of how wonderfully everyone responded with love to Larry. The irony is that if he could have found the strength to acknowledge the gay part of himself, the experience he dreaded most — exposure and rejection — would not have happened. I know he was aware of our love for him, and I trust he learned that it didn't matter to anyone that he caught this disease by loving men.

Blood Ties

LOUISE RAFKIN

"**S**IX DOLLARS OR SIXTY, you spill *something* on it!" Mrs. Evans dabbed with a damp napkin at the vague brown taint of coffee which spotted a corner of her daughter's collar. The cream silk blouse was purchased by Mrs. Evans at the local women's wear shop for Ana, her daughter. Ana stood stiffly enduring the assault.

"There," she added with a last swipe at the stain, "I think we caught it in time. Go outside so it will dry."

Ana shuffled out the screen door onto the patio. The glare off the white concrete stung her tired eyes. Her father whistled through his teeth as he arranged folding chairs in a semicircle before a small table covered with vases full of freshly cut flowers of all colors and kinds. Nearer to the house was another table draped with a sheer yellow cloth on which glasses, plates and forks caught the sunlight and sent it shooting around the large suburban yard like tiny lasers. A swingset rested on rusty paint-peeled legs alongside the garage.

"Your mother's got me onto that," her father said, pointing towards the swingset. "Wants to put in a hot tub back there. Good for my arthritis, I suppose." Ana nodded. "Want to help with the rest of those chairs?" he asked.

They unhinged the remainder of the chairs without speaking. Her mother could be heard on the phone from inside the screened porch. "I'm wearing my blue linen suit, Marge," she said. It was her mother's too cheerful voice, familiar and hollow. "Your gray dress always looks nice."

Mr. Evans went into the house to change clothes. Ana sat down and waited. Small crescents of sweat started to appear under her arms.

"Reverend Stevens is here!" Her mother's head poked out the screen door. "Come on in here, Ana, he hasn't seen you in years."

The memorial service was over in less than half an hour. Reverend Stevens offered up a few readings including sheep and shepherds and green pastures. No one cried, not even her mother. Hardly anyone had seen Jim in years. After the service, the guests ate sparsely from plates of cut lunch meats and pastries. At 4:00 the sun lost its power and slipped behind the house, leaving the patio in shade. Everyone left except two sets of aunts and uncles. Ana escaped to the bath, where she lay for over an hour until her fingers shriveled like sour grapes. From inside the bathroom she could hear the men talking about plans for the hot tub.

Fred, Ana's high school boyfriend, had called and suggested dinner. Eager for any excuse to leave the house, Ana drove her parents' two-toned Cutlass down the center street of the small town in which she grew up.

Jim had died over a week ago from what her parents and relatives believed was pneumonia. Less than two years apart, they had grown up together, riding skateboards around the hilly streets, surfing the ocean's waves on planks of hard-packed styrofoam. Together, they had developed the game of "rush hour." Crouched over an imaginary steering wheel, they screeched up and down the sidewalks, even though the only rush hour traffic they had experienced was what they saw on TV's Adam-12. When Ana was nine, they had started selling lemonade on the divider of the wide street that ran in front of their house and twisted down to the beach. Their selling price of two cents meant their mother lost more on supplies than they made in their eight-hour selling days. Jim had saved his earnings for golf clubs, Ana saved her share for a horse.

And in high school they stopped being friends. Though it was true they lived together and shared the same bathroom, their childhood partnership dissolved quickly into same-sex friendships and sibling rivalry. Jim joined the golf team and spent most of his afternoons on the golf course or the driving range. Ana took up field hockey and strove to become popular with what she saw now as only moderate success. She did what she thought was expected of her: cheerleading, parties, made the best of her mousy brown hair. For a while she dated Fred, a football player.

Jim's blond, blue-eyed good looks made him likable. And it was Jim who got the most attention from their parents. Jim's golf game warranted more dinner conversation than her straight-A report card. Her father had come close to becoming a golf pro himself, before the war steered him in another direction.

One warm night, near the end of her junior year, Ana had planned to meet Fred at midnight on the beach nearest her house. After the house had quieted, she snuck out her bedroom window. The walk to the beach seemed longer at night, the tunnel under the train tracks blacker. Her footsteps took on the proportions of a giant. Her feet sunk deep into the cool sand as she walked toward the lifeguard tower — the rendezvous. Hearing noise to her right, she looked into the thick brush to see Jim, bare-assed and bent over what seemed, in the moonlight, a male body. Jim saw Ana as she turned back running for the tunnel. Brother and sister never talked about this chance meeting; Fred called in the morning to say that he hadn't been able to escape his parents' home.

Once Jim went off to college, he rarely revealed anything personal about himself. Ten years ago, Ana had came home one Christmas to tell of her relationship with a woman; Jim watched from a safe distance. Mrs. Evans had cried. Mr. Evans refused to speak with Ana for over a week. Then he had called the family doctor to see if Ana could be changed. Finding no scientific hope, he threatened disownment if she told anyone outside the family. Ana now lived in a small, Victorian apartment in San Francisco with her lover, Alice, and their two dogs. Her parents had never visited her, never asked about her roommate. During the yearly holiday visit, she often tried to talk to her mother about her life with Alice but she was always met with silence. Both parents politely asked about her job, her dog, even her investments, but never her home life. And in every letter and phone call home she heard about Jim, his golf game, his position at the country club in Florida, his success in tournaments. And she heard in her father's voice an echo of the words, "Why can't you be normal like Jim, for christsake?" — words he had spat out to her years ago after her announcement.

Her anger at her dead brother was ugly. After coming out to her parents, she wrote Jim at Harvard, expecting some acknowledgment. He never dated in high school and seemed to enjoy the company of men, especially older men, to that of women his own age. In letters, he frequently mentioned the name of a girl he was dating. Ana thought back bitterly; he saw how it all came crashing down on her head and swore off risking his place as favored son. In Florida he made a lot of money, could rarely take time to visit home, kept his private life secret like a double agent. She had called him once or twice in the last few years, but he was always distant and formal and polite. Inside the car, Ana felt caught in a net of complicity. Did she have to continue to carry the burden of the black sheep alone throughout her adult life as she had done as a child? When Liberace died of AIDS her mother had

disbelieved the rumors — as she called them — of his homosexuality.
And her brother was no such flaming queen.

Jim's "roommate" had sent flowers to the memorial, lilies splashed
with orchids, a strange mix. Ana had received a phone call from him
three months ago at her apartment. Andrew was a golf pro at another
club and had been living with Jim for five years. His calling her was
both touching and pathetic. He rang at 3:30 in the morning, crying,
hardly making sense and obviously drunk. With the gravelly voice of a
middle-aged man, he mumbled that Jim was going to die. "We thought
it was just the flu," he said and slurred a few endearments as if she
were Jim and not his sister. Then, abruptly, he had hung up. On Monday morning Ana found a flowered notecard in her mail from Jim saying he was sorry for Andrew's inconveniencing her and that he was
feeling "just fine." There was a P.S. on the back of the card: "You've
made your decisions, let me make mine." It was the last thing she had
heard from him. A few times she had called his apartment and left
messages on his answering machine. The last time she had called, two
weeks ago, Andrew's voice was on the tape: "Thanks for your calls;
Jim's having a hard time getting back to everyone, but he appreciates
your best wishes. He should be home real soon. Please leave a message
with the date and time you called." Polite and formal even in the face
of death.

Fred had made a dinner reservation for 8:00 and already it was
8:30; Ana drove down the one-way road to the beach. She sat on the
low bluff overlooking the shore. In the moonlight, she could see the
white foam of the waves tickle the darkened sand, and between the
waves' slapping and sliding she could hear music in the distance. The
star of a bonfire lit up the sand down the beach; faces shone orange in
its glow.

Ana sat for over two hours, her mind drifting to her home in San
Francisco then, abruptly, being reeled into the tangle of family ties. In
many ways, she had given up hope for a reconciliation with her parents. Insisting on the curtains of propriety to continually cloak their
lives, the Evanses had made certain there was no room for truth in the
family drama.

It was cold and late; the distant bonfire had died down and Ana
could no longer see faces in the halo of its light. She brushed herself
off and got into the car. Driving on the well-paved streets, she noticed
that the picture windows in the suburban houses were all well lit, the
curtains wide open, shrouded in TV glows. In the city, in the

neighborhood where she lived, curtains were rarely open — even in the daytime — and iron bars covered most of the windows. These opened suburban curtains were deceptive, Ana thought, showing only carefully choreographed scenes. Bright windows as opaque as they could be. Ana drove up her parents' drive and, using the Magic Genie, opened the garage.

Mrs. Evans was cleaning the kitchen, wrapping casseroles left by relatives. Ana sat at the breakfast counter. Hearing someone in the shower, she knew it to be her father.

"Fred called, an hour ago. He said you were to meet him at 8:00. I was beginning to get worried." Mrs. Evans' voice reflected a tone of formality underscored with the expectation that Ana would detail the last three hours of her life.

"I didn't feel like going," Ana said, reminding herself of her thirty-three years.

"You should have called Fred back and told him, dear. That wasn't very considerate of you. He was worried about you." Her mother ran the garbage disposal before Ana could answer. When it stopped, Ana spoke to her back.

"Do you really believe that Jim died of pneumonia?" she asked.

The shower stopped and the hot water heater kicked in, sending a slight shudder through the house. Ana could see her mother's face reflected in the window above the sink. Her lips were drawn tight, pinched as a bird's beak.

"I don't know what you are getting at, Ana, and I don't think any of that matters now. We will all miss Jim very much."

"But you know as well as I do — " Ana was cut off by the turn of her mother and the missiles of anger directed from her cold eyes.

"It would kill your father," she said. Then she softened, daggers drawn back, and continued slowly and deliberately, "It is really none of your business to go probing into Jim's private life. And we have the medical reports."

Her mother turned back to wipe the sink, two, maybe three times more. Then she set the sponge down. Ana's legs felt weighted to the floor. Unable to move, she felt the blood leave her fingertips, drain from her head.

Mrs. Evans brushed past her daughter as she left the kitchen, not meeting her eyes. The dishwasher started to churn with a low hum and Ana turned to see the door to her parents' bedroom close. The blue-green light from a television escaped from beneath the door.

Living Day to Day — For so Long

ELAINE CAMPBELL

Elaine's husband Sean died of AIDS in November 1987. Sean, one of the estimated twenty thousand hemophiliacs in the United States, had been treated with Factor VIII, a blood product which has since been discovered to have been contaminated with the HIV virus. The following is based on an interview by the editors which took place on January 30, 1988 in Oakland.

I T WAS 1983 when Sean heard on the radio that the AIDS virus could be in the blood supply. He figured that if it was in the blood supply, then it would be in him. When you have hemophilia, you know that you aren't lucky and you don't trust chance. He called some of the blood companies, but they didn't want to talk about it. He even tried to speak to various doctors, but everybody said, "Don't worry about it, it's a gay disease."

A year later, there was talk that blood products might be contaminated. But it was just glossed over. At that time there had been only three cases of hemophiliacs with AIDS reported, and they were all possibly members of known risk groups. "Don't worry about it," was the message, "and keep treating yourself with the blood product as much as you want."

We weren't married yet, and I was willing to let it slide. If the doctors weren't worried about it, why should we worry? But Sean said, "If gay people can pass this disease sexually, why can't I? We won't get married." We went to the hemophilia treatment center to get information. When we started talking to the doctor about sex, he became embarrassed, turned red and said, "Don't worry about it."

But Sean didn't leave it at that. We got an appointment at an AIDS clinic in San Francisco. That was a slap in the face for me, my awakening to reality. We walked into the waiting room, and there were six or seven young men in different stages of the disease. They measured Sean's T-cell count — that was before the antibody test had been developed — and the results seemed O.K.

Sean was still worried that he might have the AIDS virus. During the consultation at the clinic, the doctor tried to allay Sean's concerns. He went over to the sink and turned on the water faucet and asked, "When you go to the bathroom, is it the same consistency as this water?" And Sean answered, "No." And then he asked, "Do you have problems walking?" And again Sean said, "No." And the doctor just said, "You don't have AIDS."

We wanted to know about safe sex practices in the gay community. The doctor talked about the differences between the anus and the vagina. He suggested that gay men transmit the virus while having anal sex because of the fragility of the rectal lining. Now I know for a fact that the lining of the vagina is also thin at times. When I mentioned this to the doctor, he looked at me and said, "Oh, I never thought about it." Overall, their attitude was that we should go on our honeymoon and have a good time.

We decided to use safe sex practices anyway, although not all of the time. There are the gray areas when it's unclear just what is safe and what isn't. But when you're dealing with hemophilia, and arthritis stemming from hemophilia, and then knowing about AIDS, your libido becomes quelled anyway. There were times when I equated sex with death, and later, after Sean's AIDS diagnosis, sex meant not being able to have children.

We weren't ready to have a family then. But for my birthday present in March 1985, we were planning to try to get me pregnant. These plans came to a halt when Sean was diagnosed with pneumocystis in January. The month before Sean was diagnosed, he came down with a terrible case of flu and diarrhea. Despite all of our research and awareness, we refused to relate it to AIDS. Looking back, I think Sean may have had ARC symptoms as early as 1982. He hadn't taken the test, although, if our pregnancy plans had continued, we both would have taken it. Since Sean's diagnosis, I've taken the test several times, and have tested negative consistently.

We were both very bitter about the diagnosis. We had worked so hard to dig for information and had taken as many precautions as we could. It seemed completely unfair. For instance, Sean had cut down his use of the factor — he went without it for two months. This meant that we had to curtail our activities, since without treatment Sean had severe problems with his joints.

Sean was diagnosed in Minnesota, where we had moved from our home in California so he could go to school. He had been working as an orthotic technician in the same hospital in which he'd spent a lot of his childhood being treated for his hemophilia. He wanted to get a degree as an orthotic practitioner. Sean was seven months into his degree program when he got sick and was diagnosed with pneumocystis.

I was in a fog when we were told about Sean's diagnosis. I didn't pay attention to anything around me. I stayed with Sean in the hospital every night. I quit my job as an occupational therapist and lived there in the hospital. The first night I couldn't leave — I just crawled into bed with him. They came in the next morning to draw his blood, and there I was. Sean said, "Please don't disturb my wife, she's trying to sleep." He was in the hospital for five weeks, and when he got out, he finished school. When we returned home to California he had his credential as a clinical orthotist.

Sean's former supervisor at the children's hospital had promised him a position once he'd finished school, but the administration didn't want a hemophiliac with AIDS working there. Because his supervisor rallied for him, he got a temporary position without benefits. Luckily, we still had my Blue Cross insurance from my last job.

Six months after he had been back on the job, he had a review, and they wanted to extend his temporary position for another half year, again without benefits. Because Sean had grown up in the midst of medical bureaucracies, he knew the territory and how to fight for what he needed. He went to the hospital pharmacy and told them, "You've been really good to me during all these years, and I'm sorry I can no longer buy my blood product from you since I won't get any insurance benefits from my job at this hospital. I am also going to call all the hemophiliacs who buy their blood products here and ask them to switch over to the pharmacy I'll be changing to." The next day he got a phone call from the administration telling him that they'd changed their minds, and they would give him insurance.

He was pretty healthy during the first six months, and he worked a lot. But during the last four months of his life, he couldn't work. Once he had been away from work for more than ninety days, he could no longer be an employee or receive benefits. His co-workers donated their sick leave so that he could go on being employed. A month after Sean's death, I went there to visit some people. The supervisor, who was the spearhead of all this, had converted this extra time to cash, and presented me with a check for $8000.

My family helped us out a lot through this crisis. My father rushed to be with us the same day I called from the hospital telling him about Sean's diagnosis. My mother came out later and stayed for four weeks. And my brothers and my sisters-in-law were supportive too. My family from redneck Texas told all my redneck relatives that Sean had AIDS, and they sent us get-well cards, money, and called us.

It was necessary to develop an extensive support system to keep it together, to keep hope and some meaning in our lives. I might have gone out of my mind or even committed suicide if it hadn't been for all the support groups and our friends. We each tried to protect the other from our fears. We were both such good soldiers, such strong, courageous people. Everybody said so, and after a while I got sick of hearing it.

We worked so hard, processing more in twenty months than most couples do in twenty years. We first started getting emotional support from the adult hemophiliac support group once a month. Then we started going to the ARIS support group once a week. (ARIS is a San Jose-based support group for people who are HIV-positive, diagnosed with ARC or AIDS, and their friends, lovers, and family as well as others involved with issues regarding AIDS.) We also went to a marriage counselor, and then both of us got individual counseling. No wonder I couldn't hold down a full-time job.

I had reservations about attending ARIS meetings. I was afraid that everyone there might be really sick and I didn't want to see it. Also, since they were all mostly gay men, I thought they might discriminate against women. I didn't want to be the only woman, since we are already so isolated when dealing with AIDS. I was also afraid of confronting my anger. I thought I might be really angry, and blame them for contaminating the blood supply.

Sean and I were clinging to each other when we walked into our first meeting. I joined the significant-others group. It was an incredible relief to be there. I soon realized that all of us in the group had similar needs and problems, since we were all caring for a person who had this disease.

Besides the group facilitator, I was often the only woman who showed up. There were some things that were missing for me. For instance, I was a woman going through a mourning period over losing the children that I would never have with Sean. That was hard for the others to understand.

Our group was so heavy; we were either laughing or crying. People would come in, and just let it out. We were all actually carrying a double burden — both our own and our partner's. And the roles change. For instance, I was not just the wife and friend, I also had to be a nurse, a counselor, an AIDS expert, a dietitian. When Sean was no longer able to go to work, I also had to shoulder the financial burden. And on top of it, I wanted to be with him and have some quality time together.

And sex. I was the first one in our significant-others group who finally brought up the topic of sex in the group. I kept on wondering, "Am I the only one around here who's not getting it? Does everybody else really enjoy safe sex?" I had to shake it out of everyone. Nobody had yet talked about this aspect of our relationships, even though we were all well-read on the subject.

After a while, all this obsession with what is safe and what isn't just sucks. I would get tired of fondling. Sometimes it was just terrible, and I thought, I want to get the old man on top and get it over with. But with safe sex, you can't do that. Other times it would be really great, because we went slower, which gave everything a special quality.

Sean was hospitalized and close to death six times in twenty months. I would sit down with him, and ask him, "Is this it?" Then he would recover and go back to work. He just amazed people. He had an incredible fighting spirit and really wanted to live. He wasn't the type to feel sorry for himself or to sit around waiting for death to come.

In December 1986, we moved into a one-bedroom apartment. It was nice until Sean got really sick. Home health care nurses started coming in, with IV equipment and all the other medical supplies; there was no room to breathe. So we got a house, and a woman who had been my roommate before moved in with us. We had known each other, and we knew about each other's bad habits. And Sean was comfortable with her, which was important.

At that point Sean was experiencing what the doctors diagnosed as dementia. He had gone through an emotional breakdown, was subsequently hospitalized, and was on anti-depressants. He needed a safe, quiet place. He couldn't handle people coming in, not even the nurse. The ringing of the phone was too much for him. He couldn't stand listening to me talk on the phone, even though I needed to talk to people. He became very introspective and didn't communicate much. I think he was very angry at the time, and he was wrestling with accepting his death. He was getting really tired of fighting.

Sean died in the hospital. At the end he was hardly talking, but he was so gracious. He allowed people to feed him or massage him, and he accepted it with such grace. It wasn't as if we were administering to him, it was as if he was administering to us. He wasn't angry any more, nor was he fighting. He was accepting whatever was coming.

At Sean's memorial ceremony, people couldn't believe that I was so high, in such a state of joy and ecstasy. I was celebrating Sean's physical release, his new spiritual life. Then I had to get some distance — I couldn't even look at pictures of him because it hurt so much. And to come home and live in the house without him was really hard — everything reminded me of him. I couldn't think back on the good times. I just kept reliving his last day over and over.

I still go to my ARIS group meetings to get the support I need. The original significant-others group has become so large that we've had to split it into several groups. There are now four or five mothers of sons with AIDS, as well as some female friends and sisters of men with AIDS who participate.

I've continued my work in the hemophiliac community, doing AIDS education. The hemophiliac medical community has been in a serious state of denial regarding AIDS. The National Hemophilia Association has played into it. They didn't even talk about sex and AIDS until 1985, and by then it was already too late for lots of people.

Before Sean became really ill, he and I were known as the local safe sex "experts" in the hemophiliac community. For instance, one young couple came to us and we just pulled out boxes of condoms. Months before that, the girl hadn't even known that her boyfriend had hemophilia. Lots of the young hemophiliacs deal with their disease in this way. They can just go to their room, shoot up factor, and nobody has to know. They had not been using safe sex techniques. The girl found out about her boyfriend's hemophilia, and had seen something in the news about hemophilia and AIDS. But their concern with precautions came too late. The girlfriend was tested, and she was HIV-positive.

There was another woman I'd met before we went to Minnesota who was also having unprotected sex with a hemophiliac. She was scared, but she didn't think that she could force him to use a rubber. I've learned that when it comes to people and their intimate relationships, you can't tell them what to do. It doesn't work. Since that time, he has come down with AIDS, and she has tested positive.

Some couples in which the husband is HIV-positive practice safe sex until pregnancy is their goal; then they are willing to risk the infection of the woman and future children. Other couples with an infected male partner, including Sean and me, have tried a safer means of conceiving. We tried this about five months after Sean's diagnosis. His semen sample was spun down and separated — the white blood cells from the semen, and the semen from the sperm. Then the sperm was tested to see whether the virus was present. If it had not been, we could have tried artificial insemination with the tested sperm. But since Sean was sick, he was becoming infertile. We never got to the point where there was a big enough sperm sample to test. It was very frustrating for both of us.

Throughout Sean's illness, the invisible bond between us, our spiritual relationship which comes from the heart, remained very strong. I lost my career for a while. I lost my family. I lost my future. We had to learn to live in the moment. When people asked me if I wanted to do something next week, I would never be able to give an answer. I didn't even know what tomorrow would bring. Sometimes we could just look ahead for the next fifteen minutes.

Now things have changed again. I can say that I will go on a vacation to Mexico in one month, and in two months I'll move. I am looking into the future, making plans, and I think I can keep them. After living day to day for so long, this is a new experience.

Life and Death With Joan

JENNIFER BROWN

Jennifer Brown's lover Joan Tedesco was diagnosed with AIDS in February 1987 in New York City. In July 1987, Joan chose to commit suicide.

I WANT TO WRITE about you in the daylight. Not at night, when tears well up and my naked body is racked with grief. Not at night, close to the bed where I still remember making love with you. Not in the apartment where we lived during our three years together and where you got sick. Where you lay on the couch reading medical books to find an explanation for the rashes, the fatigue, the stomach pains, the loss of memory and the shortness of breath. Not in what was our home, to which you returned in April, just before your birthday, with its grim new furnishings: a hospital bed, a commode, a folded wheelchair and a collapsible walker.

Not in those rooms where I began to have hope that together we would learn how to live with AIDS. I want to write of you in the daytime, here by the window which looks out on a little park and the nearby river. Not in the July-hot room where I discovered you hanging from the bar above your hospital bed, dead. The room where you ended your life. The room where, a month later, I found a note from you saying, "Do move! Go to a place where you can see trees and water."

I've now moved to a place where I can see trees and water. From here I'm recalling it all, my lover Joan's and my experience with AIDS. It's been a year since she was diagnosed, and she has been dead for eight months. I keep on hurting, the same way I hurt then, but the pain has become familiar.

What I feel most is Joan's irredeemable suffering, right up to her death, the vanquishing of hope. It will never be different: that this virus was inside her, from the moment we met, and years after she'd quit using drugs; that she was damaged by unnecessary medication, that my best efforts to care for her were so inadequate; that she struggled to die, because Americans don't believe in mercy killing; and above all, the fact that Joan is dead, and we'll never have another moment together.

The months leading up to Joan's hospitalization in February 1987 were frustrating for her and confusing for me. She'd had all sorts of problems throughout the summer and fall: skin rashes, dizziness, sensitivity to sunlight, stomach pains and terrible fatigue. Two visits to a hospital emergency room produced the theory that Joan might have lupus, an immune system disorder. She spent the next five months going to a lupus clinic, only to be told in December 1986 that she didn't have lupus.

During that time I was working fifty- to sixty-hour weeks at my job as head of a women's rights organization, and Joan was giving me a great deal of support. I vacillated between concern for her and suspicion of her complaints, which seemed so vague. It was the distrust of the sick, so common among the healthy.

Joan thought that she might have AIDS, but since she hadn't used needles since 1980 or '81, I figured it was just panic. Then one night in December, a friend of ours turned to me and said, "I know this is a terrible thing to ask, but has Joan been tested for AIDS? She looks just like my friend who died two years ago." Suddenly, Joan's crazy idea that she might have AIDS didn't seem so crazy after all. And she was getting much sicker.

Of course, she should have gone to a doctor, but Joan didn't have health insurance, and we didn't have much money. She'd applied for a special category of Medicaid, called the Medical Assistance Program, which is meant for people who are sick and have no income, but don't need welfare. After five months, it still hadn't come through, so she ended up applying for welfare in order to receive Medicaid. She could barely get out of the house, but kept plugging away at the bureaucracy. On Christmas Eve she received the welfare benefits awarded to her in November.

We soon found out that a Medicaid card doesn't get you a doctor. In New York virtually no private physician accepts Medicaid. The only other possibility was a hospital clinic, but Joan didn't have the stamina for the two-day wait in the hospital necessary for an appointment. Finally, on February 1987, we went to the hospital, and Joan was admitted at once with suspected tuberculosis.

At first everything seemed wonderful there. She was in a large sunny room, her appetite was back, and I was sure she'd be well soon. The first shock came when she was moved to the Medicaid floor. There the rooms were shabbier, the toilets were in the hall, and the staff seemed overworked. Joan was in "respiratory isolation," which meant she had a room to herself. There was a sign on the door giving warnings for the handling of her blood and her bodily fluids. These marked her as a possible AIDS patient, and the staff was required to use masks, gloves and gowns before entering her room. Her room was not cleaned regularly and her meals were sometimes not delivered to her, but left in the hallway.

After five days, there was a second shock. Joan was diagnosed with pneumocystis carinii pneumonia (PCP). Then we knew that she had AIDS. I remember riding the subway back and forth to the hospital during the weeks that followed, tearful, sure that Joan would die. I'd look at thin gay men and wonder if they had AIDS too. I was terrified of the agony ahead for both of us. Some nights, I stayed in the extra bed in Joan's room; otherwise, I came home to our cats and cried. I told a few friends what was wrong, but it didn't help much.

For a while, Joan was getting better, but then the nightmare hit. We'd gone through so much trouble getting Joan medical care. It was that same care that began to destroy her.

One day when I came to visit, Joan's left arm and wrist were both rigid, her neck was contorted, and her mouth drooped at the corner. I thought she'd had a stroke. She could barely talk, and couldn't hold anything in her mouth. When she'd try to stand up, she'd fall to the floor. Something drastic had happened, but I couldn't get the attention of the doctor who was assigned to her.

Eventually, they had to take notice. During the next few weeks, as Joan lay almost immobile, she was rolled onto gurneys and taken for EEGs, CT scans, and a spinal tap — in search of the mysterious cause of her paralysis. Her inability to move, combined with the hospital's preference for putting adult diapers on her, instead of letting her use a bedpan, resulted in large, painful bedsores on her behind which never healed before she died. Joan could talk a little, and told me once that she thought she was having a drug reaction. The psychiatrist who visited her told me, in a tone of incredulity, that Joan thought something had affected her central nervous system.

Once again Joan was right, and nothing will ever quell my rage over her maltreatment. After four weeks, a young intern suggested that she might be reacting to the high dose of Compazine, a drug she was receiving to combat nausea. When I heard this, I researched the drug and found that she was suffering classic side effects. It was nothing unusual, but it had caused extensive damage. Forty-eight hours after the drug was stopped, her speech was normal again. She could move her limbs, though some joints remained immobile, and she could eat. Ironically, Joan had very little nausea in the hospital and had often refused to take Compazine. But once the drug had paralyzed her, she had no choice about taking it or not, since it was added directly to the tube-feeding formula bag.

I went once to a walk-in group for care partners of people with AIDS organized by Gay Men's Health Crisis (GMHC). We went around the room telling our stories, and people talked about their lovers' good and bad days. When it was my turn, my voice came out shaking, and I said, sobbing, "My lover doesn't have any good days. She can't move, she can't even talk to me." I remember one man's story. He'd built up a business with his lover and looked forward to a happy and prosperous future with him. In an outburst of anger, he said he didn't want to be his lover's "damn nurse." I could understand his reaction, but I had never felt that way.

I understood how much Joan needed me, and there was nothing I wanted more than to take care of her. I found that easing Joan's discomfort was more important to me than all the pressing issues and politics of the women's movement had ever been. Joan told me later how grateful she was to find me there, day after day, sitting by her bed, taking care of her. She urgently needed the care I gave, and I needed the comfort I got from helping her.

I would exercise her paralyzed limbs, and force her mouth open to brush her teeth. Out of necessity I became a nurse's aide, taking her temperature, adjusting her position on the bed, attending the pump on the ever-present intravenous line and refilling her tube-feeding formula bag. She was never incontinent, but couldn't get out of bed, so every urination involved lifting her up to place the bedpan, putting on disposable gloves to wash her afterwards, then cleansing and drying her bedsores. I would chase the nurses and doctors when they didn't answer her call, and explain to the social worker and the psychiatrist that she wanted to cooperate but was physically unable to talk.

On April 13, a week after the Compazine horror was recognized, Joan came home. Medicaid provided a nurse twelve hours a day to dress her bedsores, and a physical therapist who worked with her toward the goal of walking again. A month later, I went back to work.

Joan was home for three and a half months before she killed herself. There were some wonderful moments of great hope — when she stood up for the first time, when she began to walk, when she went out onto the staircase and climbed up and down a few steps. Joan had enrolled as a GMHC client and she had gotten a buddy to stay with her on Tuesday nights when I had my care partner group meetings. Joan was very impressed with the quality of the women she met through that organization. She was thrilled to be doing again what she did best: communicating with women, reaching them heart-to-heart.

It was a difficult time, to say the least. Joan's moods ranged from optimism to rage, and her rage was very hard to take. Nothing came easy. Joan was in tremendous pain much of the time, but would seldom take the drugs prescribed, since she was afraid she'd become addicted to them. Medical appointments required an ambulance to transport her.

Joan suffered from isolation which I didn't know how to break through. She shied away from seeing most of our friends. She didn't want them to know she had AIDS, because of the drug history behind it. She managed to establish phone contact with one other woman with AIDS, and that meant a lot to her. But when this woman went into the hospital and couldn't be reached, Joan was alone again with the disease.

The apartment became Joan's prison, its two flights of stairs were an insurmountable barrier, the close quarters and dust and traffic fumes were unbearable. I tried desperately to find a new home in a building with an elevator, but I could find nothing in Manhattan.

We never managed to get beyond the crisis stage of living with AIDS. By late June, Joan was losing her vision, probably as a result of an AIDS-related infection, though it was never diagnosed. I think it was this that strengthened her resolve to kill herself.

Joan's death was horrible and unexpected, even though we'd often discussed her desire to die. I found this message in our home a few months after my lover died: "Time to end inhumanity. We need to lobby for merciful deaths for terminally ill people on this earth. An overdose of opium, morphine, or heroin would have made mine a painless, less ugly and less violent type of death."

Her message did not surprise me. Joan had told me many times after her diagnosis that being denied an end to her suffering was the cruelest treatment she could receive.

I know this is a very threatening subject to most people. Even though death is as great a taboo as sex once was, we must start talking about our schizophrenic attitudes towards it. It shouldn't be hidden away. It was such a tremendous relief for Joan when I stopped negating her desire to die. It was *not* a relief for me; I was forced to confront the awful reality of losing her. More than that, I was forced to confront my own disrespect for her wishes.

Joan said many times to me, "No one loves life more than I do." Joan's courage meant surviving a childhood of endless abuse, taking care of herself on the streets of her native New York since she was thirteen. She refused to be buried by an addiction to heroin, even though it offered her the first escape from pain. Her courage took her beyond that because she kept on loving, herself and other women. She had found many things to live for instead of heroin. She kept a glow in her heart.

I watched my strong, beautiful, smart lover as she gathered up the courage to overcome her fear of death, as she prepared to end her own life. I begged her to stop thinking about it. Despite her condition — bedridden, weakened by abusive medical treatment and terrified of what was to come — she did not let go of her will to live her own life, and to die her own death. Suicide was not a gutless act for Joan. It took all her guts to say no to further suffering, and to say yes to death at her own hands.

Promoting euthanasia, or mercy killing, as it used to be called, does not mean we are giving up hope for people with AIDS. It means respecting each other. I don't believe everyone with AIDS will die. There are treatments that offer hope and many people who live with this disease. But why deny that some of our loved ones have no hope? They need to be helped, not shamed into silence.

AIDS is not over for me, and I hope it won't be, as long as people are getting sick with it. I'm still in my care partners group, and enjoy being with the people who have been my greatest source of support throughout all this. Now I talk less about Joan in our meetings, and am more involved with helping my friends there. I've tested negative for the virus, and am deeply grateful not to be among those who must guard their own health as they care for others.

I have re-entered the "normal world" now, in which pain is largely ignored and dying is not dealt with at all. Yet it is very important to me that I maintain my sensitivity to people and their suffering, which is something that Joan's illness and death left me with. Even more important is that Joan, my unique and precious lover, remain alive within me.

II

Women with AIDS/ARC and HIV-positive Women

THE WOMEN WHO contributed to this section make up a very diverse group. Some of them have a history of IV drug use; others had a partner who had been an IV drug user or had male homosexual contacts. The profile of women with AIDS in the United States is demonstrated by these statistics: 51 percent of the reported cases of women with AIDS are among black women, and another 20 percent are Latinas.

One of the first questions asked by most women when hearing about a woman who has AIDS or who has tested positive for HIV is, "How did she get it?" When told that needle sharing and sex with someone who shoots up drugs are among the most likely possibilities for transmission, many women sigh with relief, "Then it couldn't be me."

For many women, it is unthinkable that they could be infected by a heterosexual partner. However, 21 percent of women with AIDS in the United States were infected through heterosexual contact with a person at risk for AIDS. This shows the necessity for women to discuss sexual histories and practices with their partners. According to Lynn Hampton, a contributor to the anthology and prostitutes' rights organizer, heterosexual married men make up about 80 percent of the clients whom male prostitutes or hustlers serve. The clients as well as the hustlers often consider themselves straight — and the hustlers' motivation is the quick, easy money, often used to support their drug habits.

In the United States and in Europe, where blood screening is currently a standard practice, the number of women who have been infected with contaminated blood or blood products is relatively small. The picture is quite different in most of Africa and throughout Latin America. In those countries, screening for the HIV antibody is not systematically carried out, and many women have been infected with contaminated blood. On the other hand, IV drug use in these countries is not as widespread as in the United States and Western Europe, and sharing needles contributes little to the increasing infection rates among women.

Few of the women who are HIV-positive or who have AIDS/ARC have chosen to go public; the majority preferred anonymity. Telling strangers, even friends, about your HIV infection is a difficult step. However, all the women we contacted realized the importance of going public with their stories, since they see this book as an important tool to help other women in the same circumstances.

Going Public

TEMA LUFT

Tema Luft, of Baltimore, is a board member and co-chair of the National Association of People with AIDS. The following is based on several phone conversations with the editors in December 1987 and January 1988.

"YOU HAVE A strange lump on your neck," one of my co-workers had said. I just shrugged it off. But when I went for my annual gynecological checkup, my doctor wanted to find out what this lump was all about. He sent me to an internist, who conducted all kinds of tests. He checked my stomach, sent me to get numerous blood tests and even did a spinal tap. After several weeks of looking, he sat me down and said, "Tema, you know it's bizarre, I have no idea what you've got."

On his recommendation, I went to an infectious disease specialist. He did all kinds of blood tests again. I think he figured out pretty quickly what was wrong with me, but wanted to make sure before telling me. He said that he would test me for syphilis. I got really angry with him; why would he want to test me for something so vile?

He did an ELISA test and then a Western blot. On February 5, 1987 he called me to his office and told me that I had been infected with the HIV virus and I had ARC symptoms. During the next couple of months, I continued to hope that one day he'd call me back to tell me that he was sorry and that I was not an HIV carrier. Maybe he would say that I only had syphilis. These days, syphilis would be such a blessing. I could take some drugs and it would go away.

What was weird was the fact that I continued to be examined for six months by three doctors and none of them was able to tell me what was wrong with me. I still go to the doctor who diagnosed me; he is a nice guy, and I trust him. I prefer to go to a private doctor, rather than a big medical research institution where it's much more difficult to get personal attention.

I have Blue Cross insurance, and they pay for 80 percent of my medical expenses, including the medication I have to take. I have to come up with the other 20 percent, so I spend about $200 a month for doctors and drugs. I literally get by financially by the skin of my teeth.

Not only do I have to pay for AZT, but I also have to buy all kinds of antibiotics for throat infections.

I have to take care of myself — I live alone, and I pay $400 a month rent. In order to qualify for any social service programs, you have to be in the gutter. For Medicare you have to make less than $7000 a year. I think you are allowed to own a house, but that's it. Who can live on that? I know there are people out there who do it, but I can't imagine what it is like.

I am thirty-five years old and I have supported myself for the last sixteen years, and now they want to deplete me of everything before they help me. I can do without them. I really hope that I won't become dependent on someone else.

My family can't help. My father has lung cancer, and often he can breathe only with the help of an oxygen mask. My stepmother doesn't want me around. I have asked her several times if she would give me shelter; this is all I need, and I can take care of the rest. But she doesn't want me in her house, she says.

I've also had problems with my mother. She's always arguing with me, and I told her that I wouldn't see her unless she stopped picking fights. I can't afford to be angry and exhausted. It all started when I wrote an article on AIDS for the *Jewish Times* — at that point she went off the deep end. Until last June I used to go to the synagogue with her, but she begged me not to go there anymore since she's too embarrassed about me. I was invited to speak at another synagogue, and people from my old synagogue who were there asked me why I'd stopped coming. I think I have to settle matters with my mother before going back.

Because of me, she has had to face people's fear and ignorance regarding AIDS. Once when she was at my aunt's house, her own sister gave her a paper cup to drink out of because she was worried about being infected by my mother. Since AIDS is a fatal disease, people don't believe what they are told about how it is spread. They think that the doctors are lying to them. But if transmission was possible through casual contact, everyone would have it by now.

Before I went public, my family was very nice to me. I spent a lot of time with them and they treated me well. Now that I have gone public, they are rejecting me. I've gotten so much grief from my family, you wouldn't believe it. My brother says he doesn't want to have anything to do with me if I continue with all my public activities.

But how can I stop telling people? Women have to be educated about AIDS issues. There are so many bisexual men out there who never tell their partners what they are doing. And it's the same with male IV drug users. I want to tell every woman in this country: "Use a condom, or forget it." Every woman will have to do that. Look at me, I am the upcoming AIDS person; I don't like to say that, but it is true.

A Baltimore AIDS group, Health Education and Resource Organization (HERO), asked me to speak to some women who had contacted them for information and support. One woman had a husband who is bisexual, and she was considering suicide rather than being tested. When I heard about that, I started thinking a lot. We all need someone to relate to; she needs this as much as I do. You know the AIDS crisis is going to come to the heterosexual community. If other nine-to-five workers see that it is affecting people like them, they'll change their outlook.

Another woman had tested positive and didn't want to tell her family. A woman I knew died two weeks ago, and only her husband knew she had AIDS. And then I received a call from a social worker at Johns Hopkins who told me about a twenty-three-year-old girl who had tested positive and had flipped out. She refused to talk to anyone, but finally she agreed to speak to another woman who was in the same situation. She calls me from time to time now, and mostly she cries. I really feel sorry for her — she is so young. At thirty-five, I have at least lived my life.

I used to be really healthy and energetic before I got this. I worked out at the gym five times a week. I don't drink and I don't smoke. Now I have to rest a lot. Imagine, I'd had only three sexual contacts in the last fourteen years. I was together with one man for seven years, then with another for two years, and my last relationship lasted only six months. I think I was infected by the man I was with for two years. He might have infected me back in 1985. He was a state policeman, he had lost his job for some reason, and when I told him that he had infected me, he split. I think he is somewhere in the state, but I haven't heard from him.

I don't date anymore because I don't want to get rejected. It would take a very educated man to go out with me. I can no longer think about having children, since it's not worth the risk. Most drug research programs are excluding women of child-bearing age from their testing programs. I have told them that I'll get my tubes tied and that I'll sign any paper they want, but they are just too afraid that I'll sue them one day.

But I have contacted Senator Barbara Mikulski, who is going to lobby for me and all the other women who can't get the drugs they need to stay alive. I am willing to take anything as long as I stay alive. If I was only HIV-positive, I might think of some alternative treatments, but having ARC symptoms threw me into a panic. There is an alternative cure with something called AL-721 — pharmacists in this country can mix it up for you. It's a mixture of egg yolk and all kinds of things, but the real good stuff is only produced in Johannesburg, South Africa or Israel. I don't have the resources to take off and be treated with some of these drugs that the FDA hasn't approved yet, and I am also afraid of traveling abroad. I might get really sick overseas, and not be able to come home.

I could tell you much more about all kinds of drugs and treatment. I was taking dideoxycytidine, an antiviral drug, for a little while, and then learned that you can get brain damage from it. I think a lot about all these cures and vaccines — when it sounds as if they have found something, I get my hopes up. And then it turns out to be nothing. Right now, they have AZT, which is the only thing that keeps you going. I would like to know what they do in other countries. Here they always tell you that the United States leads in research, but is that really true?

At this point I have the feeling nobody out there will get educated about AIDS unless someone in their own family has it. I joined the National Association of People with AIDS (NAPWA) in June 1987 and in September, I was the first woman elected to be a member of the board. We also elected a Latino and a black — that reflects the changes of the last couple years.

NAPWA is mostly an advocacy organization; we try to educate and inform the public. Remember when Northwestern Airlines didn't allow a person with AIDS on a plane? We fought them. At the last convention there were over a hundred people from around the country, but there are many more members.

I am the only woman in our local group, which has forty members. I've tried to talk some women into coming, but they are all afraid that someone will find out that they are virus carriers. It would be nice if there was another woman out there who would step forward and help me try to educate people about AIDS.

There are magazines like *Cosmopolitan* which seem to be working against our efforts to inform people about women and AIDS. They published an article in the January 1988 issue reassuring women that they only needed to worry about AIDS if they really got ripped up when having sex. I sat down and wrote a letter to them right away, telling them, "Look at me, I'm an average heterosexual woman, I had regular sex with a few guys and I got it." But do you think that they'll print this letter? I doubt it.

But there are other people who are trying to do some educational work. My employer, the phone company, is going to provide educational programs for all the employees. My supervisor told me that several infected employees have recently informed the management of their conditions, and it was only because I had already done it that they dared to come out with it.

And all my co-workers, except for one, have spoken with their children about AIDS. They have to take AIDS seriously, because of me. But what about other parents? There is this strong move in the country to prevent schools from doing sex and AIDS education, and I don't think that parents are always the best ones to tell their children about these issues. So many parents prefer to keep their heads in the sand about issues of sex, drugs and AIDS.

I was even told that the power company is going to send out a flyer on AIDS with their bills. That's all very nice, but it should have happened way back in 1981. Now it might be too late. I'll even meet with a health adviser to the Reagan cabinet next week, but who knows if I'll be allowed to say anything there.

I often wonder if this isn't another Holocaust. It's just like before — everyone knew about it, but chose to just sit back and ignore it. Later, everybody will say, "Oh, I didn't know." The United States did the same thing during World War II; they closed their eyes and pretended not to see. And, of course, they are all more interested in bucks than human life. Today it's just public pressure that has made the government take notice. Who else will need to die before they are willing to do something? Rock Hudson wasn't enough, nor some members of congress. Liz Taylor, who has organized several AIDS benefits, thinks it'll take at least a very famous heterosexual woman dying of AIDS before people will wake up.

I am not famous, but I do what I can. People often say, "You look great. You don't look like you've got it." But they don't see me early in the morning, right after I have gotten up. And they don't know how much effort it takes for me to continue to be part of the mainstream. Even if I'm exhausted, I still go to work. I have the feeling that once I start staying home, things will fall apart.

I am against mandatory testing. It invades people's privacy and it's also a waste of money. All of these people screaming for mandatory testing never get tested themselves. Let me stick a needle in one of their arms and we'll see how they like that. It's more important to stop the spreading of AIDS, rather than singling out those already infected. And what's the point in knowing? I know how and by whom I was infected, and what good does that do me?

I've found that being a woman with AIDS is one thing, and going public with it is another. Before I began to work publicly as a person with AIDS, I was fairly invisible. Who would think that a nine-to-five woman worker like me could have AIDS? It's those "other people" who get it. I could be anybody's daughter, the girl next door. Since I've gone public, I've faced a lot of personal and public discrimination. I've been thrown out of two beauty shops where I used to get my nails manicured, since it's now common knowledge in my neighborhood that I have the virus.

I still don't know if it was such a good idea to go public. I bounce back and forth. There are days when I really regret it, but mostly I think I did the right thing. I hope that what I am doing will help other people. We all need to get educated about AIDS, because there is no cure for it. At this point, there is just prevention. Even though my family has not dealt with me the way I have wanted, many other people have reached out to me. I have received letters and phone calls from all over the country. That makes it worth it. But the doubts remain.

I often wonder what will happen when I die. Can this be it? All these people who break their backs to make ends meet? There's gotta be something better.

Bright Candles in the Dark

ILSE GROTH

Ilse Groth, Copenhagen, Denmark, tested HIV-positive in
September 1987 and is now in the first stages of AIDS.

The Verdict

MONDAY MORNING, JUST be-
fore 10:00, the telephone rings. The doctor at the hospital wonders,
can I come see him at 2:00 that afternoon? Yes. . .yes, of course. I put
down the receiver and stand completely still, staring at the gray sky
above my studio window. My eyes see nothing but one word: AIDS. I
have AIDS. Good God, help me. Whom can I call and ask for help?
Somebody must go with me to that doctor. I can't be alone when my
world is falling apart. From this very second, life will never be the
same. I am only fifty-four and am going to die. In four hours, I'll get my
sentence. No, I have it now — it's the call from the hospital.

I did not call anybody. Deep inside I knew that we are all alone from
birth to death, especially at the most crucial points in life. Help can
only be found in yourself, in the depths of your own life energies —
and thereby in the hands of The Big Spirit, God. . .call it what you
like. So I took the bus into town and attended a lecture at the university, as I had planned. (After many years as a journalist I had just
started the study of theology — a dream which had grown over the
years.) I do not remember one word of the lecture. But I was there with
people I know, and I had to look and act normally on the outside,
while chaos was raging inside. I tried to reason with myself that
nothing had changed since the phone call — I had been ill a long
time. The hospital staff had used all of their skill to find some
mechanical fault in my organs, but without result. The only new thing
was that my illness had now a name.

The doctor was waiting for me. I will always remember him standing in the long corridor with his arms lifted in a despairing way. I
loved him that moment for the humanity in his gesture. He was sad
and shocked, and so was I. I am a heterosexual, apparently "normal"
woman, of academic background, born and bred on the sunny side of
society. I do not belong to any of the risk groups always mentioned in
connection with AIDS. It was I who had asked for the test, at the sug-

gestion of my daughter. She had seen a picture of a very emaciated AIDS patient and found some resemblance to my skinny body. I was very slim to begin with, and in the course of six months I had lost quite a bit of weight. The doctor had laughed, but had agreed, if that would soothe me. I took the test, and I forgot all about it until that Monday morning.

The doctor, a surgeon, knew as little about AIDS as I did at that time. We stood for a moment with our arms around each other. Before we parted, he arranged an appointment with the AIDS specialist. I had to come back to the hospital at 9:00 the next morning.

I took a taxi home. The driver, a man about my age, swore at the traffic, honked the horn at every opportunity, and was irritated with the whole world. I had a strong urge to hit him and scream that he should be ever so grateful for every second of his life, but I kept my mouth shut. What good would it do? In similar situations since then I have reacted, but calmly, without anger. Anger is out of place. Who am I to be mad at other people who act just as stupidly as the rest of us? We seem to have plenty of time to be offended by trivialities, as long as life appears to be without end.

Then What

Back home. The next problem was waiting inside the door. How do you tell the people whom you are closest to that you have AIDS? How do you tell your mother of ninety-two that her one and only child is ill with the most feared illness of our time? Your daughter at the other end of the country? Your son and his family? And the male friends you have shared sexual joys with — people whom you unknowingly may have taken with you into this unknown land of AIDS? Have they given the virus to others? When did I get it, who have I been with, who have I therefore an obligation to warn? How shall I live with the feeling of guilt if I have drawn beloved beings with me into this hell I am in the middle of? No, I am not guilty — did not know. How could I have known? Intellectually I know that there is no question of guilt. But emotionally. . .

As it had happened so often before, I was helped in getting started. One of my good, but not intimate, friends — one who is not in my "risk zone" — called.

"How are you?"

"Fine, thanks, I have AIDS." The words were said for the first time, the feeler sent out — five hours after the verdict. He reacted beautifully.

"Can I come around and be with you? Call me any time."

He followed up on his promise with numerous phone calls and visits — they were not empty words. Thank you, my dear. Thank you, all of you, who have stayed with me all the way. You are bright candles in the dark, you fill my days with warmth and make them rich and full.

At that time I worked in the public relations department of a big, semi-government-owned company in Copenhagen. I decided to tell my boss next, since I had to get used to the word AIDS before I could call my close friends. His first comment was something like: "Oh, shit." It became worse a few days later. He asked me, on behalf of the company, to keep my illness a secret. He knew I had written some articles in the newspapers about the bizarre situations one could experience in Danish hospitals. "We have never had anyone like you [i.e. someone with this taboo illness] in the company. It would create panic and if you come back to your job, your colleagues will look upon you as leprous and be afraid to come near you." This was honest talk, but also shocking. Was this really the attitude of the average man in this country known worldwide for its free sexual habits and its liberal attitudes?

I felt on the edge of a vast crater of ignorance, and I experienced the condemnation of everything that is outside of conventions. I was horrified to think of the reactions that homosexuals and drug addicts must encounter in this so-called humane society. When well-educated people like my boss, a trained journalist, can react so stupidly and with so little humanity, I could well imagine the more paranoid reactions of less educated people.

No, gentlemen, I will not live anonymously. On the contrary, I feel an obligation to tell my story and in my own small way help tear down the wall of taboos regarding AIDS. The wall built on the belief that AIDS is only the problem of people who do not live "decently." How close are we to being gathered in camps where we can do no harm to ordinary, well-behaved citizens? And this is Denmark in 1987.

My mother, no, I could not tell her. Not yet! I had to know more about AIDS and my situation. When I finally told the truth, she was (as I could have foreseen) admirably calm and sensible as always. In fact, she had suspected AIDS. . ."You are so skinny." Ninety-two years old and so open-minded, so strong. When my father died six years ago, in the middle of the night, she sat alone until morning with a pot of coffee and her indispensable cigars. Only in the morning did she call me. Maybe she wanted to be alone with her mind concentrated on the man she'd loved and lived with for more than fifty years.

The children were, of course, shocked, and reacted as differently as they are. My daughter had long ago cut the umbilical cord. We have been through year-long, bitter fights, screaming, crying and even laughing. They have been fruitful for both of us and left us both more mature. Today we share a warm love based upon knowing and understanding each other. We have set each other free of the past.

She wept, swore at fate and came rushing to Copenhagen to be with me, to see with her own eyes that I did not look as if death was just around the corner. She told her friends and teachers in high school the truth so they could understand if she would sometimes react a bit strangely. She wrote an essay in class describing her fear of losing me and her fear of not being strong enough to help me. In other words, she got it out in the open, where feelings can be dealt with.

My son was just as unhappy and immediately started an inner process of repression. I suspect that he has not broken the umbilical cord. (Can it be, in general, that it is more difficult for boys?) Anyway, we have never, ever had a clash. He has a wife and two children, and right now I am closer to his wife than to him. Our relationship has always been good, but alarmingly calm. He seldom calls me, never visits, even though he lives much closer to me than his sister, and he does not talk about me at home. I guess that in his way he is beseeching some unknown power by denying that I am ill. I suffer with him, and at the same time I am helpless. I can see the trauma that he is heading toward. What happens when I am gone? Will he feel guilty, feel that he deserted me? How can I tell him that his reaction is O.K., that we all have to react in accordance with our personal strength? It is not a question of his not loving me, but of not being able to live out the love; suddenly I am no longer immortal, as mothers tend to seem in the eyes of their children.

My son's reaction has become the most difficult aspect of dealing with AIDS. It's as frightening as the fact I had to face when I first was diagnosed: I might have damaged other people fatally by passing on the virus. But there is a difference, since a simple test could show whether any of my lovers was infected. Thank God, the men I have shared the good times with all tested negative.

Since then, they have told me that this shock gave their lives a new dimension. They are relieved and grateful that catastrophe was avoided. Trivialities have less importance. It's more important to avoid AIDS in the future, especially since they have seen how easily it can come from an unexpected corner.

And they are closer to me than ever, with a more profound understanding of my situation. They have seen the face of fear. They have almost met the man with the scythe. They tend to forget about him as time goes by, but they have sensed him and they understand that he is my constant shadow.

Me, Myself, I

The first weeks after the verdict I spent in a rather euphoric state of mind. Friends came and went; the telephone rang; my head was full of words that came out in an endless stream. I was very energetic, strong and calm. It was, in fact, a relief to have a concrete illness. For many months I had been through examinations, but without results. I'd known all along that I was ill. The doctors knew it too, and they'd searched for cancer, but the answer fluttered until that small portion of blood was analyzed.

I immediately started collecting all the information available on AIDS. The female specialist in the hospital, a straightforward and open woman, answered my countless questions as well as she could. For one thing, AIDS is still so new in this country that the doctors have had scant experience with it. In fact, I had more help and received more information from the AIDS-Lines, a national hotline and referral service, which is open to everybody. Most of the people working there have AIDS themselves, and/or have had personal experiences with friends in different stages of the illness. They take the time to talk over everything, something few doctors are willing or able to do.

The hospital offered me treatment with AZT, which I refused. I know enough about the side effects of AZT to make this decision. It will be the last choice when it is clearly a question of life or death, and maybe not even then. To me life is more a question of quality than quantity. I preferred an alternative treatment and my own life energies to keep me alive. So I turned down the AZT, and didn't hear from the hospital for a long time. I thought that I was of no use to their statistics, because I had turned down a treatment that the doctors have to try on the human body in order to see how it works. But that was not the case. Much later, when I contacted the hospital again, they were as interested as ever — and they wanted to know about my alternative treatments. The doctor said to me, "You are so independent, we figured that you would come to us in case you needed anything." Fair enough.

I have chosen two alternative treatments. I started seeing a naturopath who stuffs me with vitamins and minerals. I also see an anthroposoph who treats me with different medicines, among them mistletoe. At least I know that none of the medicines I'm taking can do me any harm — no unexpected side effects. There are signs that they are helping. My body has been able to fight off several colds and flus; my immune system is still working. Due to a stomach infection, I have been in much pain. The ordinary doctors could not detect it; later it was diagnosed by my anthroposoph using a special blood-crystallization test carried out in West Germany. Now the pain has decreased, and with this my optimism is returning.

Admittedly, there have been times since my first euphoric period when I felt the man with the scythe was a bit too close. Through long nights I have cried from fear, not so much fear of dying as fear of how it will happen. Will I be strong enough to leave this life with dignity, with my mental integrity intact? Will the pain become so strong that I'll have to take pain killers, with their negative effects on the mind? Am I ready to die? Will I be able to go without anger? Is my faith in God strong enough to carry me though the process without panic?

During the long nights I have also raged against God, blaming him for showing me the beauty and excitement of life. Over the past years, my joy and wonder over life's many aspects had been constantly growing, and then . . . poof, it is taken away. I've blamed Him for letting my dream of studying theology come true and then, the next moment, taking my strength.

Since the first day, I have chosen to cope with fear and rage alone, even though I can call the ones closest to me for comfort. But it is important for me to get down to the bottom of fear and to conquer it all by myself — as I did as a child when the moon terrified me. Every time there was a clear moon, I went to the room behind the kitchen and looked at it, alone and shivering. That's how we first became acquainted, and then friends. As my shadow and I are friends today.

My balance is restored, except for one loss. I miss my sexual life. I do not like my body because it is sick. I shudder at the mere thought of sex, because that is the reason, the origin, of my illness (probably a short intermezzo with a beautiful musician five years ago). But I miss sexuality as the wonderful expression of affection and love that it is. I feel poor because I cannot give and take one of the best gifts of life.

Still, I have days of extreme happiness. I have others that I call neutral, my half-moon days. But every day starts and ends in thankfulness, a feeling of being totally privileged. Privileged to be alive and able to enjoy all the small things in life. The reflection of the sky in a drop of water on a grass straw. The joy of life in a child, or a dog. The beautiful, clever words in the vast number of books to be read. Nature's changing moods. Music. And most of all, the love and tenderness I'm surrounded by.

I'm also privileged to have been shown that life is not unlimited, that it is imperative to take every moment, all of life's ups and downs as a gift. Life should never be taken for granted.

I feel reborn. For the first time in my life, I am allowing myself to be me — the best I can. Now there is no longer time for masquerades. No time for trifles. No time for politeness which comes close to dishonesty and makes me say yes, when I want to say no. No time to do anything because I feel I must.

Sometimes the nice, well-behaved girl in me asks: Is it fair to force the people around you to accept all that has happened to you, that you and only you draw the limits in your life? Yes, answers the newborn, not only fair but the most fair. At long last you give everybody the best you can give — the real you. Without withholding the negative sides out of fear that people you love might not love you. In my mind, that new way of life is the only basis for giving and taking love. Without acceptance of each and every person (including oneself) as an outstanding individual, there is no true love, no fertile friendship. Me, myself. I give you my truth and will gratefully share yours.

Just Getting By

J. H.

*This is based on an interview conducted by the editors on
January 22, 1988, in San Francisco. J.H. lives with her daughter
Sher in a small residential hotel room in the Tenderloin.*

MY EIGHT-YEAR-old daughter
said, "Mama, it's true, I heard this conversation." She had overheard
my niece talking on the telephone, telling someone that I had AIDS
and that I got it because of IV drug use. I talked to the guy whom my
niece had the conversation with, and he confirmed that she said this
— in the presence of my daughter. Sher, my daughter, said to me, "I
know what IV drug use means — it means you use needles. But you
aren't gonna die, Mama, I know it."

That all happened last week. Sher knew that I was sick, but I hadn't
told her everything. Then, when we were at the hospital last week, she
told the doctor that she was having trouble with the kids at school. I
didn't know that they had backed away from her. They were saying to
her, "Your mother has AIDS."

Sher is still my little baby. She sleeps with me. She was telling her
doctor these things, instead of me, to try to spare my feelings. Deep
down inside she's saying, "If my mother has this and the kids won't
play with me, maybe I will get sick if my mama touches me." She usually talks to me about everything.

Sher has been going to the hospital every two weeks, getting medicine. All of this illness is not fictitious, but some of it is. They think
that because of my sickness, she is copying my symptoms. She has
more aches and pains than a ninety-year-old lady.

I guess the kids found out her mama has ARC because I was on a
video-taped program for the TV news about Open Hands, an organization that provides daily home-delivered meals for people with AIDS
or ARC. I didn't think the tape would say that I have AIDS or ARC.

I also have a son, who is eighteen. Someone from Community Outreach got him a job with California Conservation Corps. Now he has
an apartment. I can't help him. See, I did a year in jail, and when I try
to tell him anything, he says, "You did a year in jail. I'll do what I want
to do." He has no respect, and I won't have him around me. I say, "I'm

still your mother, you do as I say, not as I do." We all make mistakes in our lives.

Community Outreach has been working closely with him. They have been giving him a lot of help because they feel that if I should get AIDS and die, this is the only person who can take my daughter. And they are doing great, better than I can.

My husband is in and out of trouble. He's not the kind of person who I want keeping my child. Right now he is in jail. There is no guarantee that he will be out of jail long enough to take care of her.

My income from AFDC is $460 per month for me and my daughter. I get $57 worth of food stamps a month. My rent here, for this one room, is $400 a month. That leaves me nothing to spend. It's really hard.

Right now I can't pay my phone bill. The AIDS Foundation can't help me with this. I have ARC, but I don't have AIDS yet. The AIDS clients get more than we get. They are eligible for a fund at the AIDS Foundation where they can borrow money. Since I have ARC, I get a bag of groceries once a week. They bought my telephone for me. But this month I need help with my phone bill, because I can't afford to lose my phone. It's a necessity, because if something happens to me, my daughter may need to call someone to get help.

People who have AIDS are eligible for a certain amount of money that the people with ARC are not. Why do they wait until people are deathly ill before they help them out? The people that have ARC should be eligible for the same help that people with AIDS are getting. We get sick, we have problems like they do. I have ARC. I can't work. Why shouldn't I be able to go for the money when I have ARC? Why do I have to be sick in the hospital with AIDS before I get the help? I need it right now.

I need a real support group — someplace where we can sit around and plan for our kids, our family needs, something to help us with our sickness. I want to work with people so others won't catch this shit. We have to put our heads together to teach these kids just what is going on. The people outside still haven't learned a damn thing about AIDS. They have the same fears about being around us. It's frustrating. I want to do something constructive.

My daughter is my inspiration. She's what is making me fight and hold on. She's the one who makes me think of the groups I could start to help other people. I can't give up, because I'd like to see my daughter get older.

My sister has AIDS and cancer of the stomach. They gave her one year to live. They know if she dies of AIDS, it will really affect me hard.

It'll be hard on my daughter too. My sister is getting very paranoid, as if everyone is doing something to her. She is trying to move into my building. She had a problem and ended up in the psychiatric ward in San Francisco General. When she got out, they put her in the Folsom Street Hotel [an AIDS residential program]. She is the only female there. She should be close to me so I can help her out. I'm not so sick right now. I have my aches and pains, but nothing that I can't deal with. The medication they give me helps. And they give me vitamins, but I forget to take them.

I don't have any complaints about San Francisco General Hospital. The AIDS ward started out with all men. Now they are starting to get females. Before they didn't have sanitary napkins, because everything was for men. Now they are trying to get things more together for women.

I first took the [HIV antibody] test while I was incarcerated. Since they were giving the test, I offered to take it. When the doctor called me to give me the results, he was literally crying. We had been close and he hadn't thought I would catch this mess.

I don't know how I got infected — if I was with someone, or used drugs, how can I know? I had a blood transfusion a few years ago. How many people know how they got it? I was an IV drug user, but I was always cautious how I used my works.

I've been living here for two months. If I could get another place, my daughter could have her own room. See that nice bike? Someone gave her that for Christmas. She can't ride it here in the Tenderloin. She needs some place where she can play outside in the evening. I've got an application in for other housing. All I need is my daughter's birth certificate, which costs $11. And I don't have that. I've been doing as much as I can do, but everything takes money and a lot of energy. A lady in the Salvation Army helped me to fill out these housing forms. They got me running around getting together all these forms and papers. When my daughter gets home at 4:00 — that's when I finally sit down.

I try to help other people. I put my heart into this. If I can do this, and help someone else, I feel like I've accomplished something. I've developed quite a few friends who admire and appreciate my opinions. If people want to come by and talk and find out what is going on for women like me, I'm glad to help out.

Being Positive Is Positive

ELISABETH

IF I WAS THE heroine of a nine-teenth-century romantic novel, the day that dramatically changed my life would have been dark, with an oppressive atmosphere and a thunderstorm approaching. But, since I am a quite unheroic woman of twenty-nine, living in modern Berlin, it was a beautiful, sunny April day in 1986 when my boyfriend Jan rushed into my apartment, collapsed on a chair and said, "I am positive." He had had these strangely swollen lymph nodes for more than a year, and because no doctor had been able to find the reason for this phenomenon, we finally thought of sending him for an AIDS test — just to make sure it was not AIDS. The idea that he could be infected was removed and unrealistic. This was the disease of homosexuals and drug addicts, not people like us who had just a few same sex experiences. Imagine how shocked and unprepared we were when all of a sudden AIDS was there: in my apartment, in my boyfriend. . .and in me?

In those days, the general belief was that only 5 to 20 percent of those infected would eventually develop the disease, and I tried to console Jan by telling him that chances were limited that he'd ever get the disease. Apart from that, all we had to do was to use rubbers, which we had been doing anyway during the "dangerous days," so we'd be able to handle that. It took me hours, days, and weeks to understand the full range of consequences — the first being that very likely I would also be infected.

A letter I wrote to a very close friend during the days when I was waiting for my test result shows how I felt then:

> The threat of being infected has been poisoning my life for the past three weeks. I am more or less resigned to the fact that I have been infected, as we have often slept to-gether while I was menstruating. Whenever I don't have to concentrate on something else, my thoughts revolve around

this problem. It means that my sexual life will become much more complicated and inhibited, that intercourse will only be possible with a condom and that oral sex and deep kissing will be dangerous as well. It means that I'll be carrying the stigma of the infected, and that I have to tell every future sexual partner about it. But those are only minor problems compared with confronting the facts that I may never be able to have children and that I may die much younger than I had imagined.

Over the past days I've handled this problem as if the positive result has already been verified, and it will be a relief to know for sure. There is nothing worse than this state between fear and hope. I trust myself to be capable of handling the situation and dealing with all the consequences, maybe even turning it into something positive. Right now there is a deep sadness in me and I am writing this with tears in my eyes.

I spent the whole day yesterday wondering what it means to me that I may die during the next five years. On the one hand this is a very abstract thought, and on the other it is a question that touches my deepest emotions and instincts. It makes me look back on how I have lived so far, and I realize that I have been content with my life. I don't think I've missed anything essential or that I could have gotten further in my personal development if I'd done things differently. That's a very consoling thought.

I thought I was prepared for the result being positive, but when I actually heard it, I felt as if the rug had been pulled out from under my feet. I cried the whole afternoon, night and the next morning. Then I tried to pull myself together because my mother was coming to visit me. More than anything, I didn't want her to know. I am still convinced that she'd worry herself to death.

Before, when I would have occasional nightmares, I'd wake up and be relieved that it was just a dream. Now, after receiving my test results, it was the other way around. My life became a nightmare from which I could escape only by sleeping and having nice dreams, only to wake to the horrors of reality. I felt doomed; I saw my life like a play on a stage with a background that had always been bright but now had turned to gray. I've always loved to dance; dancing for me is an expression of life and joy. But after finding out that I was infected with AIDS, I couldn't dance for months, since I felt much closer to death and sadness than to the joy of life.

I felt like a prisoner, whom the infection had deprived of the freedom to develop in any direction she'd choose. I had to stop smoking and lounging for hours in the sun. My sexual life became very restricted at a point in my life when I had finally come to enjoy sex after years of fears, inhibitions and dissatisfaction. And I felt that the infection forced me to commit myself to my relationship with Jan, because no healthy man would ever run the risk of being with me. It seemed that the only alternative to staying in this often difficult relationship was to be on my own, and this didn't appeal to me.

I had to realize that the free will that we human beings are so proud of is very limited, with the final limitation being death itself. Apparently it wasn't for me to decide when and how I would die. To preserve an illusion of freedom of will, I fled into thoughts of suicide: If worse came to worst, I could still decide myself when I'd die, instead of leaving it up to this malicious virus.

Confronting dying and death is probably the most difficult part of dealing with AIDS. In the summer of 1986, a study by AIDS specialists in Frankfurt was published, stating for the first time that probably 100 percent of the HIV-infected would develop full-blown AIDS. One of my friends, who is a doctor, and someone from the Berlin Aids-Hilfe (AIDS Assistance) confirmed this information. That's when I entered the worst phase of my depression.

Now I no longer believe in statistics. I am very angry that HIV-positive people, whose health is fragile, are deprived of any hope. This attitude might really kill them. Instead of telling people to prepare for their deaths, they should be encouraged to activate the incredible self-healing energies that each of us possesses. This is only possible if there is hope and a strong will to live.

Many cancer patients as well as AIDS patients have far outlived prognoses that were made on the basis of statistics. And even if our modern medical science hasn't come up with a treatment for certain diseases yet, it doesn't mean that nobody can be cured from such a disease. Experience has proven that there is no disease that kills 100 percent of the people who have ever gotten it. There are always exceptions. And why shouldn't everybody try to be an exception? A book by Bernie S. Siegel, *Love, Medicine and Miracles*, has encouraged me to develop this perspective.

Dealing with the question of death, I have found books by Elisabeth Kübler-Ross very helpful. She describes death as a mostly beautiful transformation from one state of existence into another. In our society, death is a taboo subject because it is seen as the end of the one precious life that one has. To me the Buddhist and Hindu idea of reincarnation and karma makes more sense than the notion of this being the one and only life and death we have. Not that I am especially happy about the idea of having to go through all of the problems and suffering of life again, but it puts things into a different perspective. Modern science has now started to reconfirm theories of reincarnation by studies of death and dying, or experiences of former lives, under hypnosis. Still, I am aware that this is a question of belief which many people might not share with me. All I know is that it has helped me in developing a sense of inner peace and calm in coping with the fact that I am HIV-positive.

I have also thought and read about the different aspects and interpretations of "disease." In modern society, disease is an unpleasant malfunctioning of the body which has to be overcome as soon as possible. Indeed, we may harm our bodies on the physical level by not getting enough rest, or by not nurturing them in the right way. But disease can also be seen as the materialization of a conflict or problem in our emotional, intellectual or spiritual "body" which we fail to recognize and treat and which later shifts to the physical level. Once we get sick, we immediately pay a lot of attention to the well-being of our bodies, and we might start wondering why we got sick in the first place. I think a disease, or the threat of becoming sick in the case of HIV-infected people, can also be seen as a great chance to reflect on our way of life, to ask whether we feel content and balanced in the important aspects of our lives or whether we would rather change something to live more happily.

I have often wondered what I may have done wrong so that my body has had to warn me by threatening to become seriously sick. I haven't come up with any clear answers. I enjoy the process of becoming more aware of what I am doing and how I am doing it, though. On the whole, I have become much more conscious of my way of life instead of just drifting along. And I have begun to recognize ways in which I didn't do what was best for me, but rather did what people expected from me. For instance, I slept with many men without really enjoying it, just because they wanted to and I didn't have the courage to say no. (Siegel's book explains that typical cancer patients are those really "nice" people who put all of their energies into pleasing others instead of listening to their own needs and desires to be nice to themselves.)

I've also realized, while wondering why I've gotten this infection, that intellectually I've perceived the world in a very negative way, although I am a good-humored person who loves to laugh. I have been politically active for years, and by dealing with starvation in the so-called third world or torture under fascist regimes, I just didn't maintain an optimistic outlook on life and the world. I am still very aware of the horror and misery that has to be overcome, but at the same time I want to enjoy the beauty of the world. AIDS put me on this new track. As paradoxical as this may seem, knowing that I am positive, I have learned to be more positive.

The change came about last September, when I was in my most depressed phase, facing death and feeling like I had been sucked into a black hole. The telephone rang and a friend of mine told me very excitedly about a shaman who had healed a friend of hers who had cancer. This shaman would come to West Germany in November, and she urged me to go for a healing. It sounded pretty weird to me and for weeks I couldn't decide, but finally I went. Psychically and emotionally I was really worn out, and I still had my doubts.

The healing didn't change my being HIV-positive, but it changed my attitude towards life, and slowly I started feeling better. The rites, ceremonies and meditations out in nature made me feel happier, more peaceful and connected to the world around me. I felt that I was part of a larger organism. During the workshop, the shaman taught us to perceive the beauty of nature. Since then I have very consciously enjoyed the changing seasons, the color of leaves, the smell of flowers, and all this has enriched my life. I have also become aware of how much friendship and love I am given. "You have the choice: You can concentrate on the negative aspects of life and be desperate, or you can concentrate on the positive aspects of life and be happy." This message sounds very simple, but I had a very hard time getting it. I still doubt it at times. However, I think for a HIV-positive person it is a matter of survival. If we don't fill ourselves with positive energy, our immune system will lose its strength to fight the virus.

There have been all sorts of puns with the word AIDS, two of which I like. A friend once said, "Maybe AIDS means for you that it is an aid to find your way on what might be a more spiritual path." The other is, "AIDS means Accelerated Inner Development."

What does being infected mean to me after one and a half years? It means that being positive has become completely a part of me and even my dreams take account of it.

It means that I am no longer afraid of death and that by overcoming this fundamental fear, I have become less fearful in general. Once the fear of death has lost its importance, all of the other horrors seem minor. However, I am still afraid of dying miserably and with a lot of physical pain, just as I have always been terrified of torture.

It means that being positive has become a crucial and dominating issue in my relationships. In spite of my worries that I'd have to stay alone because no HIV-negative man would want to be with a dangerous monster, an untouchable, I separated from Jan. In many ways I had come to perceive this relationship as destructive, the infection being just one part of that. The separation proved to me that AIDS couldn't control my life so thoroughly that it could force me to stay in an unhappy relationship. This was a very liberating experience.

I met a man who is not at all afraid of getting infected, who reacted very calmly to my being positive and transformed me from a dangerous beast into a human being again. I have been together with him for nearly a year now. Still, the fear of transmitting the disease is there, and if my partner isn't concerned, I sometimes am.

Being positive means that my sexual life has become more difficult, restricted, inhibited, controlled. I don't mind condoms at all, but not being allowed to do other practices has made my sexual life a lot poorer and altogether less enjoyable. Telling a new partner that I am positive is very difficult for me too, since I always have to prepare myself for rejection. Learning how to handle these sexual problems has sometimes made me feel like a thirteen-year-old girl facing her first sexual experience.

The fear of being rejected, to have people get panicky and turn away from me (even if it's just a little thing like refusing to drink from my glass), has made me very selective in choosing whom to tell. This has divided my friends into two groups — those who know and those who don't. Similarly, there are two versions of my life, and often I have to make up stories so as not to betray my infection.

Finally, being positive means that I belong to a discriminated minority. This really upset me in the beginning, since I have always been integrated into society. All of a sudden I was an outcast. If it becomes known that someone is HIV-positive, this person may have problems getting an apartment, a job, insurance, medical treatment. This discrimination can destroy the roots of one's existence, which is a frightening prospect.

In West Germany, some people have already lost their jobs because of being infected, although this is illegal. And last but not least, there is a tradition in West Germany about how to deal with unwanted elements of society. Bavaria was the first, and so far the only, West German federal state to introduce discriminatory laws to control groups that are considered primarily threatened by AIDS: homosexuals, drug addicts and prostitutes. These laws were initiated by the

Bavarian Minister of Domestic Affairs, Peter Gauweiler — the son of one of the administrators of the Warsaw ghetto. I don't mean to say that this country is becoming a fascist state again; it's still far from that. But we have to be careful and attentive.

After about six months of trying to cope with the infection myself, I got involved with the Berlin Aids-Hilfe and helped to start a women's group. In this group we share our experiences, support each other, look for ways to handle the situation together. All of us have found that after the initial shock and desperation, the infection has had a very positive effect on our personal development. By sharing this experience with newcomers, I hope that we can show them that life can be joyful and fulfilled despite the infection, and maybe even more so. As a woman in the group once said, "Being positive is positive!"

Through the infection and the questions I have had to confront as a result of it, I have come to a deeper and fuller understanding of life, and I will continue on this track. The dark background of this stage of my life has disappeared, and I love to dance again — consciously enjoying that I am alive and happy.

To Have or Not to Have

PENNY

*K.N. interviewed Penny, a bank employee in London,
in January 1988.*

JUST BEFORE I went under, I was hesitating for one last moment. Did I want to go through with it? Abort the baby I had been longing for? But before I could even raise my voice, I was out, only to awaken hours later in a hospital room. I can't complain about the treatment in that hospital. They did everything without asking questions. They only wanted to know if they could keep the fetus to study it. Maybe that will help other women who are infected and who want to have kids.

The other day I heard that a seropositive woman had a baby that tested negative. And both mother and father are HIV-positive. That makes me think that I might go ahead after all and try to have another baby. It might be easier than trying to adopt one. Who would want to entrust me with a child? They all think that I'll be dead in five years.

My family doctor laughed at me when I suggested getting tested for HIV a couple of years ago, and wouldn't test me. He thought that since I was in a monogamous relationship, I was the least at risk. But I had come down with hepatitis, and had never really recovered from it. I was drained of all my energies. And I kept getting fevers. Simon, my lover, had swollen lymph nodes, and despite our healthy lifestyle, he couldn't get rid of them.

Simon and I met three years ago. It was one of these business meetings, which are so boring unless one finds someone to chat with. We started talking and discovered that we both liked opera, and so we arranged to go to a performance together. Six months later, he moved in with me. Sometime at the beginning of our sexual relationship, he told me that he had used hard drugs for a short time, several years ago. Then he got a job with a small computer company, and he became so involved with his career that he quit using drugs.

Simon's swollen lymph nodes persisted, and he decided to get tested for AIDS. When the result was positive, he was so devastated that for several days he barely spoke to me. I decided to get tested right away. I didn't like the doctor who gave me the test — he treated me as if I were a junkie or a prostitute. And when he gave me the test results, he was about as compassionate as a policeman writing a ticket. "Now that we know that you are positive, be careful. Don't have unprotected sex, and don't let anyone drink from your glass." I was so stunned by his attitude, I didn't even ask any questions.

I left his office with tears pouring out of my eyes. I went to my sister's — she and I are real close — and I stayed there for several hours. I was obsessed with the possibility of my imminent death. My sister pretty much convinced me that I wouldn't die right away. We also decided not to say anything to my parents as long as I was doing fine. They are already worried enough — one of my brothers had been in a car accident some years ago, and had received several blood transfusions. The newspapers are full of stories about people — innocent victims, they write — who were infected with blood transfusions.

I decided to take off from work for a few days. Since I've always loved movies, but have never had enough time to go to see them, I went to three or four shows a day. I guess I was feeling a need to see as many as possible before dying. Then I took my credit cards and went shopping. I bought a new computer and a VCR.

That's when Simon and I started having outrageous arguments and he almost left me. He thought we needed to save all our financial resources in case one or both of us would get sick. But taking care of one's health includes taking care of one's state of mind, and I needed to please myself; otherwise I would have gone mad.

We sat down and had a long talk, and we decided to get as much information as possible in order to learn how to live with our new circumstances. We called an AIDS hotline, told them about our situation and just threw all kinds of questions at them. I didn't quite understand why we were supposed to use condoms, especially since we are both positive. But they explained to us that we could possibly infect each other over and over again, which could have serious consequences.

We had a great sex life until we both tested positive. It was really quite difficult to use those rubbers. But since we didn't want to give up on sex, this was the only choice. They really offend my senses, and putting them on turns me off. It always seems to take ages before I'm back into the swing of lovemaking. I also like the physical sensation of receiving the sperm of the man I love. Maybe that's all linked to the fact that I want to have a child.

A couple months later, we went on our planned vacation to Spain. It was early spring, and there was plenty of sunshine. Being away from home improved our relationship, since there was nothing to remind us of the danger hanging over our heads. And we said to hell with it and made love every night without using condoms. Somehow I knew that I had gotten pregnant. After I skipped my period, I got a pregnancy test, which proved me right.

I called my sister and we both were happy. I didn't tell anyone else. I think something warned me to be cautious. I went to my gynecologist, who knew that I'm HIV-positive. She told me to go see an AIDS specialist to talk about my pregnancy. The specialist outlined all the possibilities, which were all horrifying. Not only would my state of health worsen, but, most likely, I would have a seropositive baby. She told me that I could do what I wanted to do and she would go along with my decision.

I went back to my gynecologist, whom I have known and trusted for years. She was the one who helped me come to terms with my situation. Nobody told me that I had to abort, but they all hinted that it would be safer. Of course, I could have taken a chance, but I don't like to tempt fate. Right now there are days when I regret having had the abortion, but in the end I think that it was all for the better.

Living on Substances

MARGARET

Margaret is a twenty-five-year-old Viennese woman who is HIV-positive. She was interviewed by Ute Phielepeit, who met Margaret while working in a drug rehabilitation program.

I GREW UP IN a small, rural town. I went to grade school and junior high in the same city. When I was fifteen, I went to a larger city nearby and stayed in a boarding school. There I was introduced to drugs for the first time. It was only hashish, no hard drugs. At some point they kicked me out, because I belonged to a group who ran away all the time. We strolled around, went to local bars and got drunk.

First I returned to my parents, but when I was sixteen I left for Vienna. I earned my living working odd jobs. I lived in different places, and then I went off and traveled for about half a year.

I was first introduced to hard drugs when I was nineteen or twenty. It was through a friend of the boyfriend I had then, with whom I was living. I liked those people. At the beginning I idealized them, surrounded them with myths. They were so unusual. I always wanted to be different, but I never knew how to go about it. I think that was passed on to me by my parents. They used to tell us that we were something special. They didn't like it when we socialized with other people. The family just sat around all by itself, and we were bored.

We started out sniffing, and then we started to shoot up because it was cheaper. I liked to be turned on, to float; it was a bodily high.

I had no opinion about what I was doing. I pretty much gave up working, and I started to ask my parents for money. As time went by it became more and more difficult to find money. I was together with all these guys who were wheeling and dealing; every day there was something illegal going on. Some of my friends died, others ended up in jail. I was fed up. I no longer wanted to be involved with my friends' business. I wanted to earn my own bucks, and I decided to turn some tricks.

I went to Felberstrasse [an area for street prostitution] and walked up and down for a couple hours. Finally someone stopped and I climbed into his car. He drove us to a parking lot. He stopped the car and put his hand between my legs. I was so scared, I screamed out loud. I couldn't take it. I wasn't cool enough. The man just brought me back to where he had picked me up.

I got sick from shooting up. I had hepatitis, and then gonorrhea, and then my teeth got really bad. I was worried about my body and I wanted to stop. Shooting up had lost all of its appeal for me. I felt horrible and so did everyone else I'd been hanging out with. What I liked about it at the beginning had long disappeared. I stopped doing it. I drank opium tea for some time, and then I started drinking.

During that time, I had a friend who helped me a lot. He took me for hour-long walks through the forests and he talked with me. Those discussions were essential to my recovery. I haven't done anything for more than two years.

In May 1986, I found out that I was HIV-positive. The people I knew I'd shared needles with had tested positive. I went to the Aids-Hilfe (AIDS-Assistance) to have the test done. Later, when I had an abdominal infection, I went to a government clinic and I was tested again — this time without my permission.

I had considered getting tested for a long time before I finally did it, and at that time I did it in order to protect other people, not myself. Today I would do the test for myself, in order to protect myself and to take care of my health. Without knowing it, I probably infected many people by sharing needles with them.

The test result didn't come as a shock. I expected my positive results. I had a long time to get used to the idea of testing positive because so many of my friends were already living with that. And for some reason or another, I was kind of euphoric. Since I had gotten off of drugs, I thought I could handle anything. I was sure that I would never get sick, and I didn't feel threatened.

Now I see the virus as a threat because I can see it working slowly. Some of the people I know have infections, and I have to deal with disease more. I have had two general checkups. The first time everything was all right, but the second time my white blood cell count had dropped. This really upset me. I've read a lot about alternative healing methods, and I see a homeopath regularly. She has worked out a special treatment for me to deal with the virus, to strengthen my immune system and to get rid of the toxins in my cells.

I take about twenty different medications a day. I don't have much faith in Western medicine, but I don't dare depend totally on homeopathy. I'm very afraid of dying. I'm worried about being helpless, being sick and needing to go to the hospital. I have some hopes for conventional treatments, such as Retrovir (AZT).

During the first year, I didn't think much about being positive. Now I live with it all of the time because of the medication I'm taking and the health food I'm eating. I'm more cautious, especially concerning diseases. I think it's unfair that I'm positive now, after I have stopped shooting up. I'm also angry because again I'm depending on substances — this time medications — after I have gotten off the other substance.

When I got my test result, I wanted to get sterilized immediately. I wanted to do something to punish myself. I was frustrated and I wanted to hurt myself even more. I didn't do it, but I won't have children, and I regret that from time to time.

In the beginning I never kept the fact that I was positive a secret. My circle of friends is pretty small, and most of my friends are also positive. Almost all of us used to be into drugs. Those who aren't positive know that it could have happened to them too. I used to tell people that I'm HIV-positive when I first met them. And most people reacted quite normally. There was one guy who really became hysterical when I told him. He had invited me out to dinner and I told him, because I thought that he might want to sleep with me.

Nowadays, I've stopped telling people that I'm positive. Often people become overly polite, and I don't want anyone's pity. I especially don't want my parents to know. They've complained long enough that my brother and I made them unhappy. I don't want to burden them further.

In the past I used to go home with men when I was drunk. I've stopped that, of course. My current boyfriend is also positive. He has already been sick once. He does a lot to take care of himself: pressure point massages, tai chi and bioenergetics, practices that help him regain and balance his energy.

At first we didn't use any rubbers when we were screwing, but then we began to think that we might be infecting each other over and over again. Before, we would start making love, would stop for a while, talk to each other a bit, and continue later. That's impossible with rubbers. Once the rubber is on, you have to complete the act.

I'm worried that it won't be possible to find another man if this relationship ends. But maybe I won't be interested anymore. The virus dominates one's life; other issues take a back seat.

I am not afraid of enforced government actions. I also think that the media has done quite a good job of informing people about the disease. I used to read everything that was printed in the press, but I'm no longer interested, except when it's something new — for example, reports on new medications.

At the moment, I work in a paper factory. Sometimes people tell AIDS jokes. It doesn't affect me. I don't take it personally. I often compare it with the time when I didn't know anything. Then I can understand people's reactions.

My Kids Keep Me Going

D.R.

D.R. lives with her two daughters in a one-room apartment in San Francisco's Tenderloin District. The following is based on an interview conducted by the editors on January 15, 1988.

SEE THIS PICTURE? A photographer is doing a photo exhibit about women and AIDS, and she took this while we were on a picnic by the beach. They were going to use it for a photo exhibit about women and AIDS, but I asked them not to, since it seemed to exploit the kids. There was a naked guy on the beach — that's why my daughter is laughing so hard in the picture. My youngest daughter, the one who's laughing, is six. The oldest one is ten, but actually she is about twenty, since she grew up too quick. She saw too much, she heard too much. They are both healthy; I got them tested. I'm sure they're going to have more than a few emotional problems. They know what is happening with me. They don't know I have an AIDS diagnosis yet. They think I have ARC. At first I wanted to lie and not tell them. But I knew it would be messed up if I passed away, and they found out that I knew but didn't tell them.

I figured I'd just be up front with them. The little one doesn't understand. I talk about it, but it just goes over her head. I know the older one understands, because when I try to talk to her about this, she doesn't want to listen. She just says, "I don't want to hear about it."

I'm living on welfare now. I had been hurt on a job and I told my boss I would apply for state disability, but he told me to hold off and he'd get me some insurance from the company. I'm still waiting to get worker's compensation and disability. They are just stringing me along. I thought I would have my check and would have moved by now because I really hate living in the Tenderloin.

There is too much shit going around here. My ten-year-old daughter should be able to go to the store on her own. I sent her to the store once. I watched her from the balcony. I'll be damned if some forty-year-old man didn't proposition her. I flew down the fire escape and up the street. She thought I didn't trust her, but it was that guy I didn't trust. All kinds of things happen right here outside the window. If it was just me, I wouldn't mind, but I don't like my kids living here.

This is where you are sent if you don't have any money and if you're nobody special. There are a lot of good people here, but too many kids without anyone looking after them. I think there are more resources for gay men. If you're straight you don't get the same attention. For instance, housing. They have housing for gay people. You can't get in there if you have kids. I don't know, I'd think they'd want to help people with kids first.

I just got my children back. When I was with my husband, we both OD'd on drugs. There was another guy with us at the house. When you OD the paramedics and the police come. The police started snooping around, and this guy acted like an innocent bystander trying to help. So, when the police went in the house, the kids were by themselves. If he would've stayed there with them, then I would have come back from the hospital and everything would have been fine. As it was, it took me two and a half years to get my kids back.

They went to foster homes, but my older daughter was abused there. Then we went to court to get my husband's family temporary custody, and then they fought me when I tried to get the kids back. My husband's parents thought I was having a happy vacation without my kids, but it wasn't like that. I want to spend the time that I have left with the kids. They said I was using my kids to get welfare; they thought I was bringing them into poverty. My husband's parents have everything I can't give them. I don't know, I had to think about it real hard.

I went to court and fought for them. I went on a drug program, got a job and an apartment, and I did everything I had to do. They wanted to be with me. While I was fighting for them, I didn't know I was sick. I did all I could and turned my life around, and then this happened. It's too much.

I tested positive in January 1987. I tested for the money. If I could do it over again, I wouldn't have tested. I got paid $15, $8 when you first go in and the rest when you pick up your result. The guy I tested with was real compassionate. As soon as I walked in the room, I knew he'd gotten a positive test on me.

I broke out with a real bad rash on my face that turned out to be shingles. People told me I looked like I had AIDS. I thought, "Shit, I've been using drugs all those years, maybe I do." When I went to General Hospital, they told me I was just nervous and it was unrelated. When I tested positive, I told my roommate. The guy at the test site told me to tell only my closest friends about the results. The roommate told me that if the rash wasn't off my face in two days, I had to move. I had to live on the street, in churches. So the counselor was right; I shouldn't have told. But we'd been using together for ten years, and if I came up positive, I thought she should know.

By June I had ARC. I just got an AIDS diagnosis in November. I was on AZT. It gave me high fevers and popped my eardrum. It made me really sick. I had a headache so bad, I passed out in the hallway for two hours. I was throwing up everything. Even now I haven't eaten anything for a month. I've been on a liquid diet prescribed by the doctor. One lady I know who couldn't take the AZT is small like me; maybe the drug is just too powerful. Or it might have something to do with me being on methadone. I was anemic to begin with too. Right now I'm not on any of the experimental AIDS drugs.

I've met a couple of other people with AIDS in the waiting room of Ward 86, the AIDS ward at San Francisco General Hospital, and a couple I've met from being on panels, speaking and stuff. I'm always gung-ho before I go to speak in front of people, but when I get there I talk about the wrong things first. I launch into talking about my kids, get choked up and then I can't go on. I gotta figure out how to talk.

There is not enough education about AIDS. You're either gay or a dope fiend, and who cares about those people? Why don't they have a cure? Now that businessmen and "normal" people are getting sick, they're starting to care. That's how the government looks at it. If Nixon got sick, I'm sure they'd have a cure put away for him. Not Nixon, I meant Reagan. Same thing.

My kids don't get any AIDS education in their school. That's what I want to do — to get some people together and start going to junior high schools and youth guidance centers, where the kids think they are big and bad and can't wait to get into drugs. They are the ones who need to be reached. And women IV drug users. Just because they aren't sick now doesn't mean that they aren't going to give birth to a baby with AIDS. That's who I feel sorry for — all the innocent, little kids who wind up being sick.

My girls and I got to see the Pope when he was here [in September 1987]. There were some tickets available at the AIDS Foundation and I was one of the people who wanted to go. He shook my hand and touched my forehead. Somebody, by mistake, told him that my daughters had AIDS. So he walked back and took my oldest daughter and held her to his chest. And she's looking at me, and I just said, "Don't even say nothing, just savor the moment." Afterwards a local TV news reporter asked my daughter how she felt. My daughter said, "It was nice meeting the Pope." The reporter said, "You look really healthy, like you're doing good." My daughter said, "I am." I said, "He's made a mistake, my daughter doesn't have AIDS." She just walked away, no longer interested.

I follow the Catholic religion, but I don't go to church. Maybe I should; it might do me some good. I went with my friends when I was a kid. Then I got chewed out by some priest, because I was taking the bread but I wasn't baptized. I think about religion now more, since I'm sick. I'm scared now. All these years I haven't done nothing. Now that I'm on my way out, I just hope that He knows I believe, cause I don't want to go to hell. I'm trying to clean up all my sins now, while I have the chance. Before I got sick I didn't think about this. I thought I'd live forever, or at least until ninety.

Everyone in my family knows that I'm sick, but they don't know how sick I am. My mother knows, but I can't really talk to her about my fears. She helps me a lot, and I wish I could tell her all that really bothers me without it hurting her.

My mom never gave up on me. Shooting dope for thirteen years, pulling the wool over her eyes, telling her eight times that I've quit, then her finding out I'm lying. Still, she's always made me welcome in her house. When I needed things for the girls, she always helped out. But she made sure that she never gave me so much money that I could buy drugs with it. That's understandable.

I got involved with drugs when it was a fad. When I started out, I was hanging out with what I called my "good friends." I guess I was sixteen when I started snorting it. I was afraid to shoot it. Then a guy I knew told me that by snorting it I was using three times as much as I would if I'd shoot it. I shot it and I got a warm feeling and all of my problems were gone. I didn't have to think about nothing. I could escape. It was something I liked, so I kept doing it.

When I did want to stop, I couldn't. I didn't want to tell anybody I was strung out. I was afraid. So, I just shot dope every day. When I first started out, it was cheap. I'd spend $20 every few days. Now I would have to spend over $100 just to get well. I'd spend all this money and I wouldn't get high, I'd just get normal. I started to hock anything I could. Both my husband and I worked. My income and his income went straight into our arms, minus food and diapers. Every day I went to work with a $40 bag in my purse. I would go to the bathroom and fix and then I'd work like Superman.

The only time I wasn't on drugs was when I was pregnant. I was using drugs before I knew I was pregnant with my first daughter, and I stopped cold turkey in the third month when I found out. When I was six months pregnant, I got hepatitis. They tried to convince me to induce labor early, which would have more or less killed my baby. I decided that if she was sick, I would just deal with it. But she was perfect, no detox, nothing. With my second daughter I didn't use drugs at all, except for smoking weed, which I'll probably always do.

My husband isn't sick. It's kinda strange too. He's the only person I'd slept with all those years. And we used drugs together. He was always healthy, taking vitamins and taking care of himself, while I didn't. I'd go for days without eating. I still do, I don't have much of an appetite. For instance, I caught hepatitis four times, but he never caught it. It was always from fixing behind each other. He has a good immune system, I guess, and I don't.

When I first found out I was sick, my reaction was to go out and get about $200 worth of dope, come back to my house, shoot it and say good-bye. But I couldn't because I had done all that fighting for my kids and I knew it would be a cop-out. They would just figure that I hadn't really loved them, that I'd just gone out and done what I'd done before to have them taken away from me in the first place. Now my kids keep me going. If it wasn't for the kids, I wouldn't have cleaned up.

It really pisses me off, that my kids should have to suffer for something that I have. There's a lady in the building who has two little kids. About a month ago, the girls and I were taking the garbage out, and the lady grabbed her daughter away from mine and said, "Don't talk to her, she's got AIDS." People are so childish and stupid. They think if they come near my door they will catch something. Would I have my kids living with me if it was that easy to catch?

It's different around the house with the kids because of my being sick. It sounds petty, but it's strange not having the kids drink from my glass. Even though they say you can't catch it from a glass, I don't want to wait five years to find out that you really can catch it like that. I have to be cautious about everything. I just wish I could be normal again.

No one at my kids' school knows that I'm sick. The girls know not to mention that. Last Christmas we were in the corner store. There was this old man hunched over with a cane. He was trying to get enough money to buy some wine. My daughter had a dollar, and he was telling her about the spirit of the season. He said, "I'm in pain, you don't know what it's like to be in pain." My daughter answered him, "Well, I don't know what it's like, but my mom does. She has AIDS." The store was packed, and I just pretended like I didn't hear anything.

My ex-dope fiend friends who know that I'm sick blame me for putting them at risk. But I don't know where I got this from or who gave it to me. I don't trip on it — which one made me sick. People have started blaming me for being careless. How do I know who I got sick from? I've used with so many people, and anyway, the damage is done. I can't stop to think who I got it from.

Nowadays, because of the AIDS scare, I'm sure that some people use bleach to clean their needles. But I also see those bleach containers they pass out for cleaning needles down at the laundry. People use them to clean their clothes, and I don't know about their needles. I do know there are people who get a new outfit every time they use, and others use bleach. It's very easy to walk down the block here and buy a new outfit for three to five bucks. We used to buy used needles for a dollar. I don't know about the free needle programs they've tried some places. It might make needles too readily available to kids. There are a lot of kids who look up to people who shoot drugs. I wish I had had access to clean needles. If needles and drugs were just available, I'm sure some people would lose their interest in them. And they'd find something else that is illegal to mess with.

If I wasn't on methadone, I would probably be using right now. The methadone doesn't get me high, but it's helped me clean up. You don't have to hustle for your money; you don't get sick. That's why I never quit — I was afraid of getting sick, withdrawal. Methadone is a legalized form of heroin, as far as I'm concerned. You just don't have to go through the bullshit. I paid $180 a month when I first went on the program. I got other funding once I tested positive.

I haven't been hospitalized for the AIDS yet. I've written a will, and I hope my kids will go to my mother when I get sick and I can't take care of them. I don't know what will happen in regards to my husband and his parents. I can't guarantee anything. I've told the the kids that if anything happens to me, the first thing they should do is to call my mother. If not, they might end up getting separated in some foster care like last time.

Writing a will wasn't easy for me. At first when it was suggested to me by the AIDS Foundation, I was against it. I still haven't accepted the fact that I am so sick. I may seem like I'm accepting this, but it's a facade. I have to keep up this face for the kids. I could sit around complaining, but it would really make it hard on them. They try to take care of me. Now I just rest a lot, and they play on their own and know to leave me alone.

The other night there was a TV news story about some new AIDS cure. The kids got up and started dancing around. I got mad at them, because I knew it wasn't true. They looked at me and cried. I felt shitty about it. They got excited and it made me mad. It's hard.

I have been having some bad headaches. The other day I just laid down on the couch with my head down. My little one came over crying and said she thought I was lying down to die. I have created a lot of problems for them, being a drug addict and having them taken away from me. And I won't even be here to help them through that. That is the only thing that I regret. But they are pretty strong kids.

III

The Professional Caregivers

THE WOMEN WHO voice their opinions in this section present a strong case for using our common sense, human compassion and our skills in helping those who are confronted with a life-threatening disease.

With the growing AIDS epidemic, professional caregivers have also been increasingly faced with dilemmas regarding their professional ethics. A considerable number of people in the field have made it quite clear that they will not treat people who are HIV-infected or who have AIDS-related symptoms. Others have experienced the limits of caregiving. They have become overwhelmed and burned out, and are no longer able to deal with what seems to be a too complex and too dangerous situation.

Many women started out dealing with large numbers of sick men, explaining that this was one of the reasons why it was easier for them to deal with AIDS patients than it was for their male colleagues, who felt personally threatened. Since more and more women have been diagnosed with ARC/AIDS, this initial detachment is no longer possible.

Besides looking at individual caretaking, the role of the caregiving system also must be scrutinized. In the United States, the largest industrialized country without a national health system, sick people have to turn to the health industry for help. This industry plays according to the rules of profit, and access to quality care varies, depending on a patient's financial resources and medical insurance.

This forces us to think about AIDS' effects on the health care system. Pessimists predict that health services will break down because of the AIDS crisis. Optimists hope that this will be the motivation for the creation of a national health system, which will provide preventive and acute care to all people living in the United States.

Most health professionals, as well as many of the other women whose voices are presented in this anthology, have strong opinions about their personal roles and the pressing needs of people with AIDS. Hopefully someday these individual perspectives can be translated into a lasting social policy.

Skills and Pills

KATE SCANNELL

WHEN I ORIGINALLY set foot in this Bay Area county hospital, I had no intention to work primarily with AIDS patients. Fresh out of university-based medical practice as an internal medicine resident, rheumatology fellow, and bench researcher, I had decided to forgo academic medicine and practice community-based general medicine in my favorite setting, a county hospital. By now, I have been working for more than two years in this county hospital's AIDS ward.

Shortly after my arrival in the hospital, I discovered that a number of beds were taken by AIDS patients. Most of them were about my age, and many were dying. Several of them had arrived in the county health care system through tragic personal circumstances attending their AIDS diagnosis, which had cost them their jobs and sometimes their health insurance. I was overwhelmed by their illness, their very complex medical problems, their awesome psychological and emotional needs, and their dying. I was frightened by the desperation of many who wanted to be made well again or to survive that which could not be survived.

I felt all I really had to offer these patients were the tools in my doctor's bag and this head stuffed with information. So it became imperative that this small offering from me be the best and biggest it could.

During the first few months of my work, I began my hospital rounds with the non-AIDS patients because so much time was involved in the AIDS ward routine. I stayed late hours without meals nearly every day so I could figure out the fever sources, treat the pneumonias, push the chemotherapy, perform the lumbar punctures, and counsel the lovers and families. Like a very weary but ever-ready gunfighter, I stalked the hallways ready for surprise developments and acute medical problems to present themselves; I would shoot them down with my skills and pills. The diseases that would not respond favorably to my treatments and the patients who would die were all my failures, fought to the end. No patient who wanted treatment died because they did not receive aggressive full-service care from me. I became such a sharp-shooter for AIDS-related medical problems that the patients with AIDS were soon gravitating to my medical service.

Some patients were so emaciated by profound wasting that I could not shake disquieting memories of photographs I had seen as a little girl which depicted Auschwitz and Buchenwald prisoners. There were young men on the ward who were grossly disfigured by masses of purple skin tumors. One of these men, who had one eye bulging forward and the other closed tight because of his tumors, caused me to have a recurring nightmare about the Hunchback of Notre Dame.

There were so many sad stories and unhappy events on the ward. I barely spoke of these to my closest friends, and I avoided telling them how I was being personally affected by all the tragedy and death. I was hesitant to be so serious with my friends, and I really didn't even know how to verbalize what it was I was seeing, hearing and experiencing in the first place.

Months elapsed in this way. One day Raphael, a twenty-two-year-old man, was admitted to the ward. He was a large, bloated, purple, knobby mass with eyes so swollen shut that he could not see. His dense, purple tumors had insinuated themselves into multiple lymph nodes and into the roof of his mouth. One imposing tender tumor mass extended from the bottom of his right foot so that he could not walk. His breathing was made difficult by the massive amount of fluid surrounding and compressing his lungs. Tears literally squeezed out from the cracks between his eyelids. He asked me to help him. I heard the voices of my old teachers who prodded me through my years of medical training — I heard them telling me to fix this man's breathing disfunction, instructing me how to decipher and treat his anemia, reviewing with me how to relieve his body swelling with medications while correcting his electrolyte disturbances. I heard these voices reviewing with me the latest therapies for Kaposi's sarcoma. Raphael asked me to help him. I stuck needles into his veins and arteries to get more information about him. I stuck an intravenous line into one of the few spots on his arm that wasn't thickened by firm swelling or hard purple tumors.

He asked for more help. I stuck a plastic cannula into his nose to give him more oxygen. I gave him potassium in his IV line. I told him his problems were being corrected and we could discuss chemotherapy options in the morning. After I left the hospital that night, feeling exhausted but confident I'd given "my all," another physician on duty was called to see my patient. Raphael asked the physician to help him.

The physician stopped the intravenous fluid and potassium, cancelled the blood testing and the transfusion, and simply gave Raphael some morphine. I was told Raphael smiled and thanked the doctor for helping him, and then expired later that evening.

I think of Raphael often now and I ask him for his forgiveness during my frequent meditations. I also tell him that I have never practiced medicine the same way since his death; that my eyes focus differently now, and that my ears hear more clearly the speaker behind the words. Like the vision of Raphael's spirit rising free from his disease-racked corpse in death, the clothing fashioned for me by years of traditional Western medical training fell off me like tattered rags. I began to hear my own voices and compassionate sensibilities once again, louder and clearer than the chorus of voices of my old mentors. Nowadays, as in an archaeological expedition, I sometimes try to uncover how I had become so lost in the first place. I envision that I got crushed under mounds of rubble that collected over the years of my intense and all-consuming medical training, during which I strove so hard, twenty-four hours a day, to become a physician in the mode of traditional Western medicine. Some of the rubble I can identify as parts of this structure: the trend towards increasing technological interventions; the overriding philosophy that competent physicians save lives, not "lose" them; the blatant chastisement of physicians who use their "sensors" and intuitive insights when interacting with patients; the taboo against using compassion as a diagnostic and therapeutic medical skill.

Shortly after Raphael's death, I assumed the position of clinical director of AIDS services at this county hospital. Subsequently, the targets for my diagnostic sharpshooting abilities became fewer and smaller. I am no longer frightened by this awesome disease and I no longer have nightmares. I cry often and stand the bedside deathwatch frequently. I have been able to communicate with patients now, when I know that I am hearing and seeing them with tremendous clarity, and when I am able to speak clearly to them with the truths I know in my heart as well as my mind. I have substituted ice cream or local bakery products as primary or sole therapy for some AIDS patients with "complex medical disease." I have officially prescribed sunshine, a trip to Macy's and massages for some patients who had no need for my traditional skills and pills.

On daily rounds, I have visited a demented AIDS patient whose intermittent cerebral flailings sometimes made him think he was back on his Texas ranch tending the pigs and chickens. For days we had discussed the problems a few of the pigs were posing and the most lucrative way to sell eggs; once we made plans to invite the neighbors (other patients on the ward) over for a farm-style breakfast. He never saw my stethoscope or a needle in his arms; I believe he was peaceful and pain-free when he died. As each AIDS patient experiences stages of understanding and accepting of his own disease and death in the Kübler-Ross scheme, I feel I have passed through similar stages as a physician in response to the entire specter of AIDS.

I am currently waddling between grief and acceptance of this disease. I am learning how to temper hope with reality. Through a long period of unhappiness responding to all the death I was seeing, I have been able to find some peace, walking comfortably, day to day, alongside the promise of my own death. And I am grateful to hear my own voices and feel the strength of my compassionate sensibilities once again. I think of Raphael often.

Women Included

MAREA MURRAY

*This article was written when Marea Murray was working as a
case manager for Project WIN, a Boston area program for IV
drug using families with children under six.*

I AM DRIVING IN a daze on a
country road in southeastern Massachusetts after another visit with
the Smiths. Emily, the HIV-positive mother of Jacob, a toddler with
ARC, was arrested over the weekend and is suicidal. She's been shooting up for three days and seems sunken both in appearance and fear.
We talked for two hours, received visits from a housing worker, the
welfare motel manager, and Emily's husband, who escapes to the bathroom when the manager asks what happened. Why did the police
show up? She is on again, an addict coping, until he is gone. Then
once more she is a fragile, guilt-ridden and depressed mother.

It is not a typical visit for me, a case manager with a federally
funded, three-year, family-focused, community-based program, serv-
ing IV drug-using parents (mostly women) and their kids under six.
This family living in a one-bedroom home is more isolated than
usual. They are far away from any kind of support. They are actively
using and sharing needles and works, preparing for their son's visits
to the Children's Hospital, where he must go for another three-day
stay in keeping with HIV protocol. They are not involved with the
AIDS Action Committee (AAC), the Boston-based AIDS organization.
They refuse Narcotics Anonymous because there are only nine people in the group. Their son is not eligible for day care or even a play
group because he is under 2.9 years, the state's dividing line for
eligibility of HIV-infected children wanting center-based care. Their
addiction may kill them before the infection.

John, the husband, is negative/positive/negative, according to tests
administered. He will not have sex with his wife, but he shares needles
with her and blames her for their son's illness. "The way people talked
when they told us that he was ill, we thought we would've buried him
by now." John says this about his son, deadpan, yet there is an implor-
ing look in his eyes. I feel helpless and nod. Later, I give them safer sex
and needle cleaning information. I also encourage Emily to obtain

the bus pass necessary to get into Boston. That way she can attend the only women's drop-in group for the HIV-concerned in New England (although in 1988 Massachusetts plans to establish ten of these groups), or to go there for the addict support group run by the AAC. The latter would be for both of them. But they have no car. No money. No motivation. They have a dying son.

This is just one family's story. The other case manager was recently assigned a woman whose young twins are HIV-positive. Her friend, who doesn't know that this woman is hospitalized with AIDS and that her children are ill, a friend with four children of her own and homeless but for the ill woman's apartment, is diapering the infected children. What can we do? We can only discuss infection control.

The people at the hospital brush off the concerns; the patient's confidentiality must be protected. If she wanted her friend to know, then she would have told her. "But," says my co-worker, "the woman with AIDS did not even know there was any need for precautions with her HIV-infected children." "They will sero-convert," says one provider. The hospital representative disagrees; "Her partner was a user, so she was multiply exposed." Then there are turf issues as well. The homeless friend, who is caring for these children, is catatonic with fatigue and depressed. "She just looked at me," says my co-worker, after visiting her. "What can I do?" she asks us.

All of our clients are HIV-infected because of current or past IV use, not to mention sexual contact or even blood transfusions which occurred during one of the many typical hospitalizations for endocarditis, hepatitis, pneumonia and premature delivery — the payback for IV-using women.

We talk to providers whose first question may be, "Has the child been tested?" Usually there is more concern for "innocent victims" than for their parents. This has always been the case with IV drug users, even before AIDS. And now? Now, we hear doctors say, "Tell them, don't get pregnant." I am a white, middle-class social worker. I appear at the door and they think I'm there to take their children away. Or I am unmarried and childless, so who am I to recommend inpatient, residential treatment? Where can a woman get that and child care as well? In Boston, there is one place, and its state funding is shaky. Another place is only for pregnant addicts.

And that is the city. There is no place to get methadone between Boston and New Bedford, near the Rhode Island border. My needle-sharing family on the South Shore, without a dependable car, is slowly killing itself. And there is no saying whether they'd consent to methadone maintenance even if it were available. My other family in Roxbury also lives with four kids in a one-bedroom home. They are ineligible for public housing's waiting list of 12,000 people because Mom has a record for possession, trafficking, simple assault. . . As she uses IV cocaine, methadone is not appropriate.

We ask ourselves if we can do preventive work around AIDS with women who are still shooting. We see them in hospitals, temporary shelters, homes where they live with male partners or other mothers. We try and put ourselves in their places, but we cannot.

Our clients deal with lack of access to affordable housing, medical care, day care, education and employment options. They also have to deal with the issues of race, sex and class as facts of life. They lack information about how to clean needles. However, while most are aware of their risk for infection through needle sharing, often they do not acknowledge the risk of sexual transmission through an infected partner. Needless to say, it's difficult to discuss sex or even needle-sharing/works-sharing risks as they deny continual, past and present IV use. Some have been tested and say they have tested negative — thus "safe."

"Making him wear a condom" is not necessarily an option for AFDC mothers, women who are hooking to feed their children and stay high. Nor is it an option for women with religious or ethnic backgrounds which look upon barriers as genocidal. Not to mention women with partners who beat them or their children.

It is considered a woman's fault if she becomes pregnant, if she gives birth to an infected or addicted or HIV-positive child. And if the child dies, if she gets sick, if her partner is infected? It is a vicious cycle, all the more for an addicted parent, an addicted mother, a woman.

I think of my white, gay male friends and the grassroots organizations which have done so much in our community. There is so much more to be done with multi-problem, drug-using families, who are dying in our major cities and outside them — from addiction, poverty, and HIV infection. We do the best we can, but there is so much more that needs to be done. IV-using families are hard enough to reach, but with HIV complicating the situation, it can be overwhelming.

On my good days, I view it as a challenge. On my bad days, I wonder what will become of us. All of us. Women included.

Confessions of an Antibody Test Counselor

JAKLYN BROOKMAN

FOR THE PAST two and a half years, I have been an AIDS antibody test counselor at the Alternative Test Site in San Francisco's Castro District. According to my latest tally, I have disclosed over 3,000 test results. About 1,000 have been positive, with gay and bisexual men being the main recipients of these. Sometimes I fantasize that I'll be given a bronzed lab slip when I give away my final result.

What have I learned during all that time? First of all, I can talk dirty now, without a flinch. I can deftly ask anyone from a pubescent male to a sixty-year-old grandfather whether he's had unprotected anal intercourse and, if so, was he on the top or the bottom?

But it hasn't always been this way. When I began this work, AIDS was rather remote from my life. I thought only gay men in the fast lane succumbed to this illness. And when I heard stories about some of the sexual practices within gay male culture, they just fueled my own biases. I felt a bit like Pat Nixon in her good, Republican cloth coat, often thinking, "What's going on here? I just don't understand these boys." I must admit, I still have some difficulty in counseling sessions when I hear about water sports and fist-fucking, but I've become more curious, less judgmental. I think of myself as Margaret Mead, entering into another culture which has little to do with my own experiences.

Upon my telling people what I do for a living, they often respond, "Wow, Jackie, how can you do that work? I never could." As though I were this other-worldly creature with a special talent most mortals do not possess. I am aware that my involvement in the world of AIDS conjures up images of death, uncertainty, and loss. I also harbor these images as I struggle to help my clients understand how to live a life of quality and fulfillment.

Why did I get involved in this kind of work? As a child, I watched my young mother's prolonged illness and eventual death from cancer, a process which was very troubling and confusing. No one in the family, including my mother, was permitted to discuss her imminent death. This made it impossible for me to comprehend her deteriorating condition. Whenever the topic was broached, most often by my mother, her concerns were quickly dismissed with a twist of humor by my father. As an adult, I realized how damaging that experience was for me, and how it must have been for my mother.

The paralyzing inability of my family to directly and compassionately acknowledge the thoughts and feelings surrounding her illness and death made it clear to me that I wanted to "do" death differently. I knew I wanted to provide an arena for the expression of all kinds of feelings, whether they be mine or others'. I also knew I needed to work through my own mounds of terror and confusion, legacies of that experience which haunted me for many years.

In light of my past, it's probably not surprising that I spent many hours poring through the works of Elisabeth Kübler-Ross, Stephen Levine, and Ram Dass, in order to gain a different perspective on issues of both life and death. As an antibody test counselor, I have been in the position of encouraging my clients to focus on enhancing the quality of their lives, while also validating the real fears and concerns about the often ominous prognosis of a positive result — most likely symptoms of AIDS or ARC down the road. This is never an easy task for me. Sometimes I feel like the Grim Reaper. Yet I see this interaction between myself and my clients as crucial. For those infected, it's often the first step in the long process of assimilation and integration of their positive test results.

Disclosing a positive test result can be both difficult and compelling at the same time. There is a certain kind of intimacy which evolves — a tender connection with these erstwhile strangers has been and continues to be a special component of my work. For many of those infected, the trip to the test site is a way to begin preparing for the future. I give my antibody test clients what I would want in the same situation: love, support and knowledge.

Along with my role as emotional support person, I also see myself as the organizer, the pivotal person who supplies information and education appropriate to their needs, no matter whether the test results are positive or negative. With everyone, I stress the importance of following risk-reduction guidelines. I want my clients to leave our session committed to accepting individual and collective responsibility to fight this epidemic.

What happens and how I feel during a counseling session depends on who is in front of me, that client's issues, and how he or she receives the test result. Sometimes I become "Jackie, the Savior," earnestly pouring out tons of information and advice in the hope that my suggestions will magically transform this person. I sit there hoping that self-destructive clients will stop drinking so heavily, stop having unprotected sex, and stop abusing themselves and their health with such regularity.

"Jackie, the Savior" also wants to make things better for the many who are grieving. It is not unusual to hear the litany of losses reeled off with anguished resignation: fifteen friends, two lovers and a best friend just diagnosed. We both sit there silently, acknowledging that it won't end here. I secretly conjure up ways to erase all the losses from the past and those that will eventually follow. Yet I know very well that just being there, at that moment, on that day, will have to suffice.

The life of an antibody test counselor is full of limitations. I can only see people once, usually for half an hour. I don't know anyone's name, unless told, nor what they will do when they leave my office. At the beginning, this was very disturbing to me, as I wasn't used to such a format. I am also a psychotherapist in private practice, seeing people on an ongoing basis, and that continuity is a significant part of my professional life. What is striking about the structure of counseling at the test site is how it so aptly mirrors the feelings many of us share who work within this epidemic: feelings of not doing enough, wanting to give more, wanting to have more information, wanting to have more time available — as if the "moreness" could somehow alleviate our feelings of sadness and helplessness.

Over the past year, however, I've begun to re-evaluate my role and its limitations, and I have learned to respect my ability to be a knowledgeable, astute, caring counselor, as enough. For the most part, I've also come to trust that those in front of me will get the support they need and will do what's in their best interests. I've learned that taking on the pain of others is not useful to them or to me. I am no longer left with the chronic feeling that I haven't done enough. I've begun to see myself and my role as but one stopover on a long journey for my client. This has helped diminish my own need to appear to be the omnipotent counselor.

There have also been times when I've been quite inspired by my clients. There are those who come through my door who have been assuming they were positive for a long time and who have already radically altered their lives for the better. Many have spoken of getting out of stressful jobs and relationships, and now they are meditating, eating well, exercising, and so on. This always reminds me that in our culture we are too preoccupied with the quantity of life rather than its quality.

It has also been a pleasure to give out negative test results to those who were sure they had been infected due to a history of high-risk behavior. I like it when I can say, "Guess what, cookie, you're negative!" I watch the varied responses, which can range from disbelief to tears of joy, thanks to God and, on two occasions, marriage proposals to me. The tone and the atmosphere in the room go through a remarkable transformation as anxiety is replaced with lively talk of plans for the future.

Even though the Test Site is mainly frequented by gay and bisexual men, the focus of the media on the importance of the test and the risk of heterosexual spread of the disease has motivated many people at low risk of exposure to get tested. At times this fluctuation in risk populations has not been easy for me. In one session, I'll disclose a positive test result to a gay man who not only must confront his own mortality but also must grieve the loss of others. My next session may be with a low-risk person who remains skeptical about casual contact not transmitting the virus and who fires off a barrage of questions: "Are you sure I can't get it from kissing? Are you sure I can't get it from mosquitoes? Are you sure I can't get it from restaurants? What about gay waiters?"

This encounter may be followed by a meeting with a single man who says, "Condoms are a drag — they're like having sex wearing a raincoat. And besides, I'm negative." When faced with these situations, my desire to maintain the stance between the patient and emphatic counselor wanes considerably. It can even come to the point where I sometimes feel downright bitchy, barely holding back the urge to say, "Listen, buddy, you're wastin' my time. There are others out there who really need my assistance." I know that dealing with such reactions is as much a part of my work as comforting and counseling those who are already infected with the virus. It still rattles my senses to be presented with this roller coaster of human scenarios.

As I've become aware that I can't "make it better" for those who are antibody positive, I've also begun to disengage from the "trying to convince" mode I find myself in with those who remain resistant to the reality of risk. I consciously try to keep myself in check so that I don't become that bitchy, impatient counselor. Sometimes it works and sometimes it doesn't.

I don't want to give the impression that all those at low risk are either difficult or hysterical. That is not the case. In fact, I've witnessed increasing numbers of men and women who are diligently taking responsibility and are committed to following risk reduction guidelines. It has been particularly refreshing to hear of the many women who are insistent that their partners use condoms. In the classic words of one woman client, "He's not gettin' near me until he puts a slicker on his puppy." Stories such as this make me hopeful that many people in this town are taking an active role to stop the spread of the virus.

Hope is an essential ingredient in doing this work. However, feeling it and conveying it to clients can be fraught with conflict and contradiction. I've often asked myself, "How can you encourage this person in front of you to be optimistic, when chances are that a host of symptoms and a life hampered by limitations lie ahead? So many are dying, have died, will continue to die. . ." But despite the harsh realities of this epidemic, I go on hoping. I see myself as a cheerleader, banking on my clients' abilities to strengthen their positive sides.

I feel fortunate and privileged to have had the opportunity to be one of the many who work on the front lines of this epidemic. Of course, it has its very unglamorous aspects, including the monotony of espousing for hours on end the virtues of condom use, the ever-threatening political climate, the low pay, and the always rising numbers of cases. Recently, my work has expanded to training others around the state in how to give test results. I like the fact that I can take my considerable experience on the road and have an impact on many more people. I hope to continue to educate and train others so that all of us on the front lines can help in dealing with an inhumane disease as humanely as possible.

A Day in the Life

DENISE RIBBLE

IT WAS THE END of a long day. And a long week.

I was sitting at my desk, pondering for the umpteen millionth time how to get a woman enrolled in an Ampligon trial (the testing program for an experimental AIDS treatment), when all the studies to date were stating that being a gay man (or at least pretending to be) was part of the inclusion criteria.

Tacy poked her head in the door and said, "Do you want to talk to someone you don't know who won't give her name?"

"Yeah, sure," I said, glancing at the clock: 6:00 p.m. Why do people always wait until late on Friday to call?

"Hello, this is Denise Ribble, the health educator at the Community Health Project. How can I help you?" I asked.

"You spoke to my friend Mary several days ago," said a soft voice. "She said you would be able to help me. I think I'm at risk for AIDS."

After a few seconds of mental sorting, I recalled Mary as an ex-IV user and prostitute who had called on Tuesday.

"Why do you think you're at risk?" I said. There was a pause. "Can you talk there? Is someone listening?" The pause continued. "I'll ask some questions and you can answer, O.K.?"

"Yes," said the voice.

"Did you ever shoot or skin-pop drugs?"

"No," said the voice.

"Did you ever have sex with bisexual or gay men?"

"I'm a lesbian. I've never had sex with a man," the voice said.

"Did you have a transfusion in the last ten years?" I asked, running through my mental checklist of possibilities.

"No," said the voice.

"So why do you think you're at risk for AIDS?" I wanted to know, running out of patience.

"I'm a vampire," said the voice, ever so softly.

114

"Oh," I said, like the frog in the wide-mouth frog joke. It was my turn to pause. A long pause — while I frantically tried to remember what I had learned from Bram Stoker, *Dark Shadows* and *Interview With A Vampire*. (I took into consideration that this was a joke.)

"What exactly are your risky practices?" I asked in my best professional tone.

"Well, when I go to the bars, I make sure I pick up women who are having their periods, and I have oral sex with them."

"Is there any way you can change your practices?" I said.

"I supposed I could drink the blood of animals," said the voice distastefully, and then continued, "If I'm really a vampire, I don't have anything to worry about because I'm immortal. But if I'm just a fucked-up woman who drinks other women's blood, I'm at risk, aren't I?"

"Yes," I said.

There was another pause.

"Can vampires donate a tube of blood for HIV testing?" I inquired gently.

"Yes," said the voice. "I already have an appointment. But I wanted to talk with someone about my real risk and what I can do about it."

"Well, for now you can change your risky practices — that'll reduce your risk if you're not infected," I explained. "And you really should wait at least three months from your last exposure before getting tested."

"And if I tested positive, can I come to your clinic?"

"Yes," I said. I had a brief flash of Catholic school fear — you know — fire, crosses (even though I've been a Buddhist for years). Then, mostly I felt sad. For this woman had not thought herself at risk. Now she was. Despite her unique circumstances, she was frightened and isolated.

Not so different from many other women I had talked to.

Crack Down on AIDS

YOLANDA SERRANO

*Yolanda Serrano is a substance abuse specialist who has worked
with the Association for Drug Abuse Prevention and Treatment
(ADAPT) since 1980 and is now its executive director. ADAPT
made national headlines in January 1988 when they announced
that they would defy state law by distributing free hypodermic
needles to IV drug users to slow the spread of HIV infection. The
following is based on a conversation with Ines Rieder on June 3,
1988 in ADAPT's Brooklyn office.*

ADAPT WAS FOUNDED in 1980
by recovering addicts and health care professionals. Although we had
differing philosophies about our approaches to this work, we shared
the common cause of defending the rights and interests of people
recovering from addiction. Currently we have about 300 members,
mostly professionals — doctors, lawyers, social workers, nurses, many
of whom have a previous history of drug abuse themselves.

By 1982, some of us began to notice an increase in the rate of death
of our patients. At that time no one was addressing the connection
between AIDS infection and IV drug use. But soon we realized that we
could no longer ignore the problem. Rather than forming a separate
organization focusing on IV drug use and the spread of AIDS, this
work became another focus for the work of ADAPT.

We have been working in the streets of New York providing education and encouraging risk reduction. We also have people who go to
hospitals and take care of those with AIDS-related illnesses. Every
week we have support groups for the ADAPT workers here in the
office.

ADAPT was the first group in the city to deal with AIDS among
drug users on a practical level. In 1987, the City Department of Health
funded us with less than $200,000. We receive some private donations,
but considering the amount of work there is to do, our activities are
very limited by our budget. Until recently, ADAPT relied on volunteers to do outreach work, but now we have some funding to hire paid
staff members, the majority of whom are recovering drug users.

Most of ADAPT's work is done in the city streets. The members come to the office to pick up supplies for distribution: informational brochures; condoms; sterilization kits which include bleach, water, cotton, a cooker (a small vessel to mix drugs); and instructions for sterilizing needles. Because of our work, people in the shooting galleries have begun to change their behavior. Now it is the drug users themselves who come to our office to pick up bleach kits, and they are teaching each other how to clean their works.

Some of our outreach workers are attempting to organize IV drug users. They teach them how to protect themselves, how to educate each other, and how to gain access to drug and medical treatments. There have been attempts to organize active addicts to prevent the spread of the HIV virus.

We have been proposing a needle exchange education program. We'll have a van going into the drug trafficking areas, staffed with a health educator, a nurse, and security. We'll engage users in short conversations, and we hope eventually they'll change their behavior. Our primary goal is intervention, not the needle. If we have regular contact with users, we can try to get them into treatment. Or, if they continue to use drugs, they will learn to use them safely.

The other goal of this program is to collect dirty needles and to distribute sterile ones. Going into some areas of New York, you can find dirty needles all over the streets, and little kids playing with them. Clean needles must be easily available, either by selling them or having exchange programs where a drug user receives a clean needle by handing in a dirty one. People see this program as condoning drug abuse, but we look at it as an issue of public health. We have to try to save humanity, and right now the virus is getting out to the public through IV drug users. There are similar programs in the Netherlands and Australia, and the legal distribution of clean needles has not increased the level of drug use.

We started out focusing our attention on IV drug users, but now crack has come on the scene, and it is as deadly as IV drug use. If you go to the crack houses in the morning, they are practically empty. They fill up in the afternoon once kids are out of elementary or junior high school. That's when business is booming. Many adolescents get their money for crack from prostitution. Once their families find out about their addiction, it's often too late. By that time, the teenagers have turned to violence, and are mostly hanging out in the streets.

There are more women addicted to crack than men; at least, there are more in the treatment centers. I have no explanation for this. In the crack houses, I've seen beautiful girls wasting away. They've lost weight; their clothes are literally falling off them. Many of these girls prostitute themselves for $2 to $10 per sexual act. There are ten-year-old prostitutes who manage to look like they are seventeen. The latest fad in the crack houses are the so-called "headhunters." These are women who give blow jobs to guys while they are smoking. Being a "master blaster," the term that refers to guys who have orgasms while inhaling crack, is the ultimate.

There are about a quarter million IV drug users in New York, and there are 43,000 treatment slots available. If someone goes to jail for drug use, it costs the state about $45,000 a year. The cost of a drug-free rehabilitation program is about $12,000 a year per person, and an outpatient methadone program costs $3,000. Prevention — that is, education in schools — would cost $500 to $600 per student a year. Catching people before they start is cheap, but society doesn't put its efforts and resources in the right place.

Many people like to think that IV drug use is not their problem, since they have nothing to do with junkies. But they would be surprised to see the make-up of people in our drug-free and methadone treatment programs. The addict is your doctor, your police officer, your bus driver. Many people go to work every day and nobody knows about their addiction. They carry this secret with them, and the fear that someone will find out about it.

That's why women are very much at risk for the virus. Somebody could be in recovery from a history of drug use, and potentially a carrier of the HIV virus, and he is out there dating. How can a woman know the history of this man? I believe you don't see large numbers of women who are HIV-positive because they are still healthy and unaware of their infection. But within a few years, this situation will change dramatically.

Of New York's quarter million IV drug users, 80 percent have sexual partners who are not using drugs. About 60,000 women of childbearing age are using IV drugs, and if they are infected, they can pass the HIV virus on to a child during pregnancy. As well, those women who are the partners of IV drug users may give birth to children who have a 50 percent chance of being infected.

We tell our women not to have babies until a vaccine is found, and that might not be for a good many years. But once they are pregnant, we tell them to get good counseling and evaluate their choices. IV drug users are often left without options. When they are on drugs, they sometimes don't ovulate, and by the time they realize they are pregnant, it's often too late for an abortion. Add to this the poor prenatal and general care they receive, and you get the full picture. I know of one family in which the woman, her husband, and two of the children are HIV-infected, and she's pregnant again.

All the statistics about AIDS are underestimated. In New York a group of researchers went back to the records of about 3,000 IV drug users who died over the last three years. They found that 53 percent had died of infections thought to be HIV-related. None of these people had been diagnosed with AIDS. They were drug users with jobs and families, and many of them had been in treatment programs. The same is true today. Most IV drug users dying from AIDS don't know it.

I think that one of the reasons for this is that many hospitals don't want to be known as AIDS hospitals. They feed their patients lots of antibiotics, take care of their infections, but they don't diagnose them. Also, if people are diagnosed, then they are eligible for all kinds of social services, and possibly eligible for AZT treatment.

I've worked as a substance abuse specialist in a methadone clinic since 1980, and twenty of my patients have died of AIDS since then; they were all in recovery trying to change their lifestyles. The husband of one of my girlfriends was infected with HIV through IV drug use, and he died as early as 1982. The husband of another friend died in 1985. Six months before he died, the doctors knew he had AIDS, but neither of them was told. She died two years later from AIDS.

Not enough money is reaching community-based organizations where most of the work needs to be done. The money goes instead to building powerful consortia and to major hospitals. We think that the money should be allocated to small grassroots organizations. We know what's happening in the streets, and we have ideas for programs that will reach people and help them to prevent the spread of the virus.

Beyond the Call of Duty

HEDWIG BÖNSCH

Hedwig Bönsch is a nurse at an outpatient clinic in West Berlin. She writes about Jochen, her first AIDS patient.

JOCHEN WAS SENT to our outpatient station in January 1986, and I volunteered to take him on. At that moment, he was only a "case" to me, and I didn't know what consequences this job would have for me. In the meantime, almost two years have gone by, and I have taken care of four AIDS patients. I have learned a lot, and I have also changed due to it.

I still remember the first time I went to see Jochen. It was a Monday; I had already taken care of four patients, and now I was on my way to him. I was uncertain. All I knew about him was that he was a thirty-four-year-old gay man with AIDS. On the way to his house, I thought, "What will he look like? What does he expect from me? Will it be possible to talk openly? Will he like me? How much help does he need? How much does he want? How will I feel when I walk away from our first meeting?"

Today, I know that he had also wondered about me, and he had asked himself, "How will I get along with her? Does she have fears and prejudices?" My name alone, Sister Hedwig (in German a nurse is addressed as sister, and Hedwig is a name that was more common at the beginning of the century), made him think that I was an older, conservative nurse. He hoped that I was nice and that I would be helpful. After all, he needed help.

I rang the bell, and it took a while until a tall, gaunt, young man answered the door and smiled at me. I was relieved. We started talking, and soon we decided to call each other *"du"* (the familiar "you"). This was new to me, as so far I'd always addressed my patients in the polite form (*"Sie"*), but I liked the more intimate atmosphere of *"du."*

I prepared his breakfast, gave him his medications, arranged his bed. He talked very openly about himself, about his childhood and about his problems. I realized quickly that he was well-informed — both about his own condition and about AIDS. In fact, he knew more than I did. Hadn't I thought I knew everything? During the following weeks, Jochen and I talked a lot about the disease. I often thought he was informing me, rather than the other way round.

At the beginning I thought that I was the stronger one, because I was healthy. He was dependent on me, he needed me. Today I know this isn't true. As a nurse, I was used to providing the physical care for healing, such as giving shots and changing bandages. With Jochen, I found out how difficult it was to do little, just to be around, to listen. This psychological care is very important for AIDS patients, as they go through stages of anger, despair and resignation.

AIDS patients are thin-skinned. Like most seriously ill people, they have antennas which register how the caretakers behave. Are we giving them our hand? Are we looking in their eyes? Are we sitting on their bed or keeping a distance? I often had the impression that Jochen was both consciously and unconsciously testing me. Are we able to handle their anger and their aggressions? Will we return despite their behavior? Or do they have to adjust themselves as patients, put aside all feelings and desires?

I concluded that occasional anger or aggression directed against the nurse can be a sign of trust: "This nurse can deal with it, I don't have to protect her/him, s/he won't hold it against me. I can do what I feel like doing at this moment." On the other hand, nurses can fight back when they have the impression that the patient has taken advantage of them. It is important that lines are drawn.

In the course of the following weeks, Jochen and I became friends. I liked to visit him, and I spent some of my leisure time with him. We were partners in a common struggle. This was a new experience in nursing for me.

When I first started dealing with AIDS patients, I talked a lot with my friends and acquaintances about my work. I think I got on their nerves, but I had to deal with so many new issues.

It was sad to realize that it was not only the AIDS patients who were isolated, but that I was, too. Few people listened to me. One AIDS patient once wrote, "When I was given my diagnosis, I thought I had crossed a border. Everyone around me was on one side, and I was all alone on the other. I could see them, I could talk with them, but they didn't understand."

I had a hard time telling people what I experienced at work. Several people retreated. One person even told me, "I won't see you again if you continue to take care of AIDS patients." Others made me feel guilty by constantly saying, "Think about your family." I wasn't used to defending what seemed obvious and reasonable to me.

Jochen's health changed often and without warning. The medications he was taking had many side effects, and I had to keep a close eye on him. After some weeks, his overall condition deteriorated. He vomited frequently and lost his appetite. He was without spark and depressed. He had fevers and dizziness and was often unable to get up. He became weaker and weaker. He knew it, and he monitored his own deterioration. There was little I could do to motivate him. When I wanted to take him for a walk, he would respond, "What for? I don't know why I should walk." Finally, he agreed to go back to a hospital.

This was the end of my job. The outpatient station gave me other patients to care for. This is everyday life.

But I couldn't leave my new friend alone, and I went to see him in the hospital every day. My family fully understood my situation, and my kids often came to the hospital with me. This was a positive experience, since kids have a much more relaxed attitude towards disease and death. We should think twice before we exclude the sick and the old from interacting with the rest of society.

The relationship between Jochen and me was one of trust and affection. I asked him to be honest with me, to tell me when I was being a bother and when I should leave. I also made it clear to him when I needed or wanted to go away. I went to see him only when I wanted to be with him and not out of any obligation. We both knew the other's thoughts and intentions, and there was no reason to pretend.

Jochen once told me something which gave me lots of strength: "You know, I like your company, because you don't expect anything from me. You are simply here and you take me as I am."

After four weeks in the hospital, Jochen's state improved. He had more strength, and he could walk short distances on his own. The herpes infection on his face had healed. He was very pleased about that. His mind was more balanced, and he looked forward to being released from the hospital.

The day he was released, I picked him up, and since the weather was nice, we decided to go for an ice cream. It was hard on him, but at the same time it was good for him. He enjoyed being part of life again. Each day was important, and he experienced it more consciously.

Besides me, Jochen's mother and an acquaintance from the self-help group took care of him. We were the only people who were around him. His mother showed up every day after work, took care of the house and the cooking. She had a hard time comprehending that her son was seriously ill. All her grief was translated into activities. She cleaned most of the time and made everyone nervous. She could not sit down and just listen to her son, and she treated him like a child. It was only at the very end that she accepted her son's death and let go of him. Jochen was often very irritated with his mother's behavior, but he didn't want to hurt her, because he needed her.

His stepfather and his sister didn't help much. His sister showed up only out of a sense of obligation, and Jochen was aware of it. The stepfather came between mother and son. He complained because his wife spent most of her time taking care of her son. He never shared her grief. She was on her own with all her problems. Her work, her daily visits to her son, and the sorrow all overwhelmed her. She needed someone to talk to and cry with.

Jochen and I often went out together. We used to have breakfast in some cafe, or Jochen would show me former work sites, or places he liked. This was always exhausting, but it was a nice change. We also watched TV together or looked at old pictures. He was hopeful and made many plans. His biggest desire was to go traveling. His mother took him to her garden, and he enjoyed being outdoors.

Jochen was still having a good time, and we had lots of ice cream together. His thirty-fifth birthday was coming up, and he had planned to invite us to his mother's garden for a celebration. I was looking forward to that, but I was also wondering what to say to him on that day, what to wish him. I decided to talk with him beforehand.

I told him, "I find it hard to say what I really want to say, in front of your family. I'll tell you now. With all my heart, I wish you courage and energy for the hard time ahead of you. I hope you'll have many beautiful hours without pain, and some time to be happy. I hope you'll have a wonderful birthday, because both you and I know that this is your last one. And I like you."

I was surprised at myself for saying this. I think that I was able to be so honest and open because I knew Jochen so well. I took him in my arms and we both cried a little. He thanked me and asked me if I was going to be with him when his time came. I agreed.

Two days before his birthday, he started having epileptic seizures. He was found unconscious and was brought to the clinic. He was in bad shape, and we were all shocked. Since he had been doing well during the past weeks, all of us had pushed aside the fact that he was sick, that he had AIDS. But reality always catches up with us.

When I came to visit him, he was depressed. He was upset, because his desire to celebrate his birthday outside was now impossible. I felt for him, but I couldn't console him. His condition deteriorated every day. He became weaker and weaker. Each week he was able to do less; he needed help for almost everything, and he changed. His memory began to fail him. He had a hard time concentrating and being articulate. There were days when he did not get up or when he refused to eat. He could no longer smoke cigarettes. They started to feed him intravenously. And everyone knew that he would never leave the clinic.

We decided to stay with him twenty-four hours a day. It was difficult, since there were only three of us, but we managed. For fourteen days we stayed with Jochen, all day and night. We all got close to one other, and even now, we see each other.

During his last days, Jochen suffered. His heart was still strong and he had a hard time dying. Like everyone else, I stayed with Jochen for many hours. I had reached my limits, and I was extremely tired and worn out.

But when Jochen died in his mother's and my presence, it was all too sudden.

I felt empty during the days following his death. All of a sudden, I had all the time in the world. For nearly three quarters of a year, I had been with Jochen every day, and I was sad.

The terminally ill have a different set of values. They remind us that we should live differently, in the here and now, with more awareness of imminent death. Many issues and problems lose their importance. AIDS makes it impossible to dream about the future. Younger cancer patients often repress the disease and its consequences. They talk themselves into being healthy. AIDS patients, on the other hand, know what they are up against. They say openly, "I'm very sick. I know that I have to die." They often plan their funerals and write their last wills.

This doesn't mean that AIDS patients are not afraid. They have less fear of death, but more fear of dying. They ask themselves, "Will I be in pain?" "Will I be alone?" "What do I still have to go through?" Some say, "If I can't stand it anymore, I'll kill myself." All patients prefer to die at home, for they are afraid of being left alone in some hospital. And they reach a point where death is seen as deliverance.

It's difficult to watch people get weaker and sicker, and to see them die with lots of pain. It is difficult to describe what it is like to take care of an AIDS patient who goes blind and who still has his death ahead of him. It is almost too much to see handsome, strong men turn into gray-haired, skinny beings, dependent on others for everything.

Nevertheless, I want to take care of AIDS patients. I think AIDS is an issue that concerns us all. Everyone can get sick with AIDS, including our children, our co-workers, our neighbors. When doing this work, I know that I am needed. Once again I was made aware of what nursing means for me, why I had chosen to learn this profession. I started questioning religion, death and my own sexuality. I reflected upon my life. What do I want? Am I satisfied? Being with someone who is dying puts me in the role of a student and of someone receiving a present. I've realized how nice it is to listen and to be silent. I've discovered new aspects of my personality. I've gained strength; I am more at ease with myself.

Exhaustion

LORNA FORBES

I AWAKEN AT 2:00 on Saturday afternoon. It is not the first weekend I am experiencing this exhaustion. Lying in my bed, I reflect upon my last few weeks as a medical social worker and psychotherapist for people who are HIV-positive, and those who have been diagnosed with AIDS or ARC.

Soon it will be three years that I have worked full time in the AIDS field, often more than forty hours per week. My first two years with an AIDS hospice in San Francisco involved caring for and losing 130 men to this insipid disease. During the last year, while working in an AIDS outpatient medical clinic, I have still been dealing with men with AIDS, but more and more women and babies require my professional services as well.

I have not moved from my bed. It is now 3:00. My body feels heavy, but my heart feels full. My phone remains unplugged. I begin to think about my female clients one by one. I start to be scared again. Can I do this? Not only are these individuals young, but they are women, and some of them have babies. Now I have three, not one, issues with which I will over-identify; I am thirty-five, I am a woman, and my yearning to have a child one day is very strong.

Two weeks ago, Susan called me. I had never met her, but she had seen our doctor when she delivered her baby. For ten months, Susan was told that she should meet me and seek help. It was obvious that she did not want to face the reality of her situation. She burst into tears over the phone and stated that she was feeling overwhelmed and didn't know if she could cope. When she came to my office, she brought her baby. Eric was one of the most beautiful babies I had ever seen. He looked incredibly healthy, and he was a happy and playful nine-month-old. Susan chose to see me by herself, while the father, her partner, watched the boy. The clinic staff told me later that he was very loving with his son.

During our first session, Susan told me that in her eighth month of pregnancy the doctor advised her to take the AIDS antibody test, because she admitted to IV drug use prior to her pregnancy. She tested positive, and was told at that time. When thinking back on that day, she remembers that it did not sink in. It was almost as if she put on blinders, not to think what this could mean for her and her unborn child. Her baby was tested after birth and was also HIV-positive. He was in an incubator for one week, not HIV-related, but he developed normally after that with no complications.

Susan became immersed in raising her baby, and although she was usually quite responsible with basic medical checkups for her son, she refused any psychological or medical help for herself. Susan chose not to tell anyone, since she didn't trust any of her friends to keep this secret. Over the last few months, she has been more isolated and more afraid. Because of the constant media splashes about AIDS, thoughts about it are impossible to avoid. Her partner of three years has been supportive, but has his own fears due to his past IV drug use.

Susan sobbed quietly as she talked about what has been disturbing for her. She said she loves her baby so much that she aches with pain every time she looks at him. Every day she wonders if this will be the day he will get ill with an AIDS infection. She fears that she and her partner could get sick and die, and what would happen to her son then? She agonizes over her guilt feelings for having caused the virus to be transmitted to him.

I picture myself in her situation. The plight of women in the AIDS crisis poses an exorbitant amount of social and psychological problems. A few months ago, one of my female clients discovered that she was HIV-positive when she was three months pregnant. Her doctor and other professionals advised abortion. I spent a lot of time with her discussing the worst and best scenarios. I told her that it was ultimately her choice and that her baby had at least a 50 percent chance of being HIV-positive. This was an incredibly difficult decision for her, since she had always opposed abortion. Eventually she decided to keep the baby, saying, "I asked God to do what is right. I prayed constantly." At six months she miscarried. This was an extremely painful loss for her, but now, in retrospect, she thinks God made the decision for her.

A few of my other female clients are HIV-positive or have ARC. They were infected because they shared needles, had a bisexual partner, or had a blood transfusion. No matter what the cause, these women face isolation, and they are afraid to tell others. There is not enough social support for them. Some of them don't tell current or prospective partners about their seropositivity for fear of losing them. The women with children, of course, are in the worst situation. Many of them are single mothers with financial worries. I have found that many of my female clients have the lowest attendance rate for medical or psychological appointments at our clinic.

It is now 6:00. I lie back down on my bed with a heavy heart. Sadness engulfs me. I am still tired. I know it is going to get worse. I drift off into sleep, my favorite form of escape.

IV

Lesbians Facing AIDS

ALTHOUGH THERE ARE many contributions by lesbians throughout this anthology, this section focuses on some of their specific concerns. Initially, lesbians were dealing with AIDS issues not because they were threatened by a disease, but rather because AIDS seemed to have a significant impact on the gay community and its political future. The first order of business was organizing health, social and support services for people with AIDS, and lesbians have continued to play an important role in this task.

At the beginning of the AIDS epidemic, lesbians' first reaction was that this new virus could not affect their lives, stressing the notion that lesbian sex is safe sex — they were protected. Now we know there are lesbians who have been diagnosed with AIDS, and there have also been reports of sexual transmission between women.

Besides these practical survival issues, lesbians have been involved in tackling the long-term legal and social implications of AIDS. The epidemic has fueled homophobic legislation, and even though these laws may be aimed primarily at gay men, they also work against lesbians in concrete ways. Obscenity laws, initiatives to restrict already limited gay educational materials, and hampering the work of AIDS organizations by labeling certain projects "immoral" effect gay women as well as gay men. Certain states have attempted to pass laws quarantining people with AIDS; other states have passed laws for mandatory HIV testing. Whenever laws like these are implemented, they first target a specific group, but they can later easily be applied to the rest of society.

What will be the outcome of these years of AIDS work? Will lesbians' visibility in the gay rights movement increase? What will be the response by gay men to the work lesbians have done? These questions have been raised by many lesbians, and will be discussed for some time to come.

All That Rubber, All That Talk: Lesbians and Safer Sex

MARY LOUISE ADAMS

Mary Louise Adams is in the editorial collective of Rites,
*a lesbian and gay magazine published in Toronto, Canada.
She is completing research on women and AIDS-related
issues in England.*

TWO WOMEN SLEEP together for the first time. As they fall into bed, there is little discussion beyond "I want. . ." and "I want, too. . ." They have fabulous sex and make plans to see each other again. Several weeks into the affair, one of the women stops going down on the other. Again no discussion. Feeling a little neglected, the other woman grows concerned. Why the sudden changes in behavior? Could it have anything to do with AIDS? Eventually they talk, and apparently it does.

Hearing this story secondhand, I thought how well it encapsulates a lesbian sexual response to AIDS. Overcoming squeamishness about dental dams is but the least of our worries. Frank talk about what we do in bed is going to prove far more troublesome.

In the last year, lesbian and gay and feminist publications have been full of information about safer sex for lesbians. AIDS groups have distributed pamphlets, such as the one from the Women's AIDS Network in San Francisco. But have lesbian sex lives changed? Are lesbians practicing safer sex?

A friend is astonished at even the mention of safer sex for lesbians. She certainly doesn't know anyone doing it. "Do we really have to?" she asks before admitting that, yes, she is a bit reluctant to sleep around these days. Another woman tells me she's stopped having oral sex while either she or her lover is menstruating. Her lover sulked for a while, but she's getting used to the idea. The two of them know a couple who do practice safer sex, but not because of AIDS; they're trying not to share candidiasis, a chronic yeast infection. I talk to a woman who's familiar with the safer sex guidelines for lesbians. She's having an affair with a woman who is just coming out, who is living and sleeping with a man. No safer sex. A woman in London who has been

130

researching AIDS and women for months breaks up with a lover and has a few little flings. Safer sex never even crosses her mind. She can't think of a single woman who does it, either. My lover has an affair with a woman I don't know. They discuss risk and conclude they're safe. I start having dreams about AIDS. Do I suggest to my lover that we do safer sex with each other? No.

Most of these women, myself included, know about safer sex, know that lesbians can transmit HIV. Some of us aren't totally convinced that the virus can be transmitted between women as easily as some sources of information suggest, but we know the possibility exists. So what's the problem? Why the reluctance to "play safe"?

In the spring of 1987, a lesbian and gay newspaper in Toronto printed an article about AIDS support counseling. Buried toward the end of the piece was a brief reference to two local lesbians who had tested positive for HIV, with no mention of how it had been transmitted. I read the paragraph twice, just to make sure. Other women tell me they did the same. It wasn't talking about New York, but about Toronto; the women were lesbians; we perceived them as part of our community. Dearly held illusions about lesbians and AIDS began to wither. A short while later, I ran into a friend. "I guess we have to start practicing safer sex," she said. "What's that mean for dykes?" I told her what I'd read. We found it difficult to imagine. All that rubber; all that talk.

A month or so after our conversation, Theresa Dobko and Yvette Perreault of the AIDS Committee of Toronto held their first safer sex workshop for women. They booked enough space for 100, but still they ran out of chairs. They discussed transmission, risk, barriers to HIV, other safe possibilities. We shared fears and fantasies, role-played pickups and other sexual situations, and we were reluctant to leave when it was over. I'd never been to an event where lesbians, bisexuals and straight women listened respectfully to talk of sexual differences. When the assorted dildos on the table in front of us were presented, quite simply, as pleasurable accoutrements of safer sex, not a single woman in this gathering of feminists raised any objections. I knew something special was happening, and learning about safer sex was just part of it. We had defined new terrain for sexual debate — at last, a motivation to tell each other what we really do in bed. AIDS created a context in which we had permission — indeed, we were obliged — to talk about sex, graphically, non-judgmentally. Women loved it.

We live and love in communities that rarely make space for the airing of sexual difficulty or difference. We subscribe to an image of effortless, unadulterated sex that's wondrous and sublime. The frustrating, the annoying, the disappointing remain our personal failures as we struggle to match the ideal of automatic woman-to-woman ecstasy, spontaneously inspired by feelings of love and tenderness. Women whose own particular practices may challenge this notion rarely speak out, and so the notion remains prevalent: lesbian sex "just happens." Safer sex, on the other hand, is premeditated and deliberate and may demand "implements." It's not the least bit mystical. For many women, safer sex is not lesbian sex as it's meant to be. Further, it's new and threatening and requires frank discussion. We're not, any of us, so good at that. Though the workshop in Toronto seemed to uncover a well of untapped potential.

Women who are experimenting with roles, fantasy and props already have experience in talking, in negotiating a sexual situation. Safer sex becomes another challenge, latex merely something new to eroticize. The task is not so much to expand constantly upon what is safe (with all the reliance on medical opinion that entails), but rather to expand upon what is sexual. For women within certain strands of feminism, this might prove difficult. Sex toys, fruit, fantasy, consensual s/m, sexually explicit stories, voyeurism, sexy talk — these aren't too widely embraced as part of the feminist canon. But with a little common sense, they can be safe. Is it time to re-evaluate?

Certainly there are women who know about safer sex, who think they should be doing it, but many of them are too embarrassed to suggest it to a new lover, or they can't bear to give up all that wetness or, believe it or not, they forget. Others anticipate unsympathetic responses from women who don't really understand what safer sex is all about. Cindy Patton, author and Boston AIDS activist, was speaking at a conference in London where she talked about a lesbian who wanted to know about safer sex. "Do you know anyone who actually does it?" the woman demanded. "Me," Cindy answered, offering herself as an example. The woman immediately reacted to her as someone dirtied. Instead of being commended for their responsible stand, people who practice safer sex are often shunned, assumed to be contaminated.

Misconceptions about AIDS still abound, many of them leading to the huge numbers of lesbians who still think AIDS will never mean anything to them or their lovers. Their hopeful thinking is encouraged by articles like the one recently published in *off our backs*.

The intent of the *oob* piece was to make clear that the people most frightened about AIDS are not the ones most affected by it, which is partly true. But the authors then suggested that lesbians are getting out of hand when we stress the importance of safer sex between women. If lesbian communities were closed and static havens, the point would be valid. But they aren't. Some lesbians do drugs, some use gay men as sperm donors, some sleep with men, and some sleep with bisexual women who sleep with men. It's nice to think that some-one will tell you her sexual history at first prompting, but that's not as simple as it sounds. Not everyone feels able to divulge details of past experiences, particularly if they contravene community norms.

And of course we mustn't underestimate the power of our concepts of "community." Many of us do feel a responsibility to keep it, as well as ourselves, clean. We can't assume any longer that we'll be mon-ogamous for life, that we're the chosen people and immune to HIV, or any of the other things we use to convince ourselves that we and our community are inherently safe.

Safer sex isn't solely about individual initiative. Those of us who enjoy a little company during sex will need the support and coopera-tion of other women for our changes to be effective — in our own sex lives as well as in the community. As more of us go to workshops, talk to our friends or write stories, safer sex will become more a part of everyday life, and it will be easier to love and play safely. Indeed, the safer sex rap group may become a preferred site for lesbian cruising. There's no reason for healthy sex to be lonely or dull.

I Am Not a Port in the Storm

MÔNICA PITA

*Mônica Pita is a volunteer working with GAPA (Grupo de
Apoio a Prevenção a AIDS — AIDS Prevention Support Group)
in São Paulo, Brazil. Before getting involved with GAPA, she
was an activist with GALF (Grupo Ação Lesbica Feminista —
Lesbian Feminist Action Group). She is twenty-three years old
and lives with her father and her sister on the outskirts of São
Paulo. Marlene Rodrigues interviewed her in January, 1988.*

Q: How did you get involved with GAPA?
A: One night in 1985, I was watching TV and I saw a report about
GAPA's activities. At that time I wasn't involved in any groups, and I
was ready to do something again.
Q: Did you know that GAPA was dealing with AIDS issues?
A: Yes, and that's what caught my attention. People with AIDS are not
only discriminated against because of their disease, but also because
most of them are male homosexuals. As a homosexual woman, I'm
also discriminated against, even more than men are, but when it
comes to AIDS, men are worse off.
Q: What was your first contact with the group?
A: I got their post office box number, and I wrote them a letter explaining that I was a lesbian and wanted to work with them. I never
received an answer, though. Then one day, during a meeting at City
Hall on Brazil's new constitution, I saw two GAPA members and told
them about my letter. They invited me to the group's next meeting,
and I went to it and enjoyed it. I liked the fact that GAPA provides not
only AIDS education, but also direct support for AIDS patients.

A while later, they called me and asked me if I could go and see a patient who was in very bad shape. I went straight to the hospital and
ended up helping with his care.
Q: How many patients have you taken care of?
A: Several. I stayed with one man until he died. He was a baker from a
very poor family, and he lived in a housing project in the outskirts of
São Paulo.

Usually I went with another person from the group, in order to
make it easier for both of us. We had to talk to the patient as well as to

the family, who didn't really understand what was going on. They had moved to São Paulo recently and didn't know many people. They wanted our support, and they also needed someone to talk to. All his friends had disappeared, and the family was quite lost.

Q: Was it difficult to talk with this guy?

A: It's always difficult to talk with AIDS patients. These people are sick; they know that they are going to die. I arrive and greet them. But I can't ask, "Are you all right?" because they are not. My biggest fear visiting AIDS patients, though, is that they might think I am a port in the storm for them, and that they might try to put all their hopes for survival on me. After each visit the patients improve, because someone outside their family encourages them to eat, to talk. And, I think, the family believes that the sick will be cured by such visits, and this really worries me.

Q: In what ways do you take care of the patients?

A: I only talk with them. All of them ask to be touched or held. Their first reaction to my visit is to take my hand and hold it firmly, and then they kiss my face to see my response, to see if I'll reject them or not.

Q: And how do you react?

A: I try to behave as naturally as possible, even though it bothers me since they are trying to test me, rather than doing something spontaneous. They want to see if I'm disgusted, because there are people who don't even want to go near them.

Q: Do you discuss these things during GAPA meetings?

A: Yes. Besides the bureaucratic meetings, there are meetings specifically for those of us who visit people with AIDS. There we can talk about the difficulties we encounter in this work. Many of us find it very difficult to deal with people without showing pity, to be on equal terms with them, since their disease puts them at such a disadvantage, physically and socially. Therefore, it's important to clearly define our limits, and not fall into paternalistic roles. Another problem arises when we have to cancel a visit. The next time, the patient is very angry and depressed, thinking that he has been abandoned. We have to explain that we have our own limits, our own lives and obligations.

Q: Besides visiting people at home, do you also go to the hospital?

A: Yes. Usually the hospital social worker lets us know which patients aren't being visited by their family or friends, and we go and see them.

Q: Have you encountered any problems dealing with the hospital?

A: At the beginning it was very difficult. Several times we couldn't even get in. The employees thought that GAPA was trying to control their work. But then we just lied, and told them that we were friends of the patients.

Q: How is it to go for a visit in the hospital?

A: In Emilio Ribas Hospital, São Paulo's largest public hospital, the only one with an AIDS ward, visiting hours are from 2:00 to 3:00 every day, and we are not allowed to enter the rooms; we have to remain at the doors. In private hospitals, visitors are allowed to visit in the rooms, but have to wear masks, gloves and gowns, to avoid infecting the patient with germs brought in from the outside. In the public hospitals, this protective gear is not available to visitors, often not even to the nurses, because of the hospitals' limited budgets. And the AIDS ward is completely understaffed, because few professionals agree to work with these patients due to their fear of contamination.

Q: What does the hospital provide for the patients?

A: A room, sheets for the bed and a pair of pajamas. Some medication is also available, but often the hospital doesn't have enough money to provide patients with the drugs they really need. In some cases, the family buys them. The majority of the patients are very poor, and often GAPA ends up buying medication for them, as well as items like soap, toothpaste, shaving cream, cigarettes.

Q: Do people accept the fact that they are going to die?

A: Oh, no. One day when I went to the hospital, several patients had just died. When I arrived, a lot of people were crying, gesticulating, screaming; it was quite a commotion. These people had not been allowed to enter the hospital because the patients they'd wanted to see had died the night before. They had not been notified by the hospital, but found out right there at the door.

When I arrived at my patient's room, he wasn't there, and I was shocked and upset, thinking that he had died too. But he had only gone out for a moment, and when he came back he wanted to know what all that noise was about. I had to lie, saying that I didn't know. My patient knew pretty well what was going on, but he wanted to hear the word "death" from my lips, instead of from his own.

This patient, like so many others, hadn't accepted that he had AIDS. They invent all kinds of excuses to explain why they are in the hospital. Whenever someone dies, they all feel very bad. The next night many of the patients don't sleep, thinking that death will come and take them away too.

Q: Are there many patients who never receive visits?

A: Yes. GAPA does its work for them, so that people won't be left all by themselves. The Brazilian government should take care of them, but instead, money is wasted on gigantic and useless projects. Money should be spent to assist people with AIDS. But since this disease is so closely linked to sexuality, a taboo subject, people with AIDS are discriminated against, and all the public campaigns are insufficient.

When I go to see people, especially in the poor neighborhoods, I realize how ignorant the public is about AIDS. Not that it's their fault; it's just that they are not given any basic information. Once on a bus, I saw a gay man sitting there and everybody was looking at him and whispering about him. When he got up and left, nobody would sit where he'd been seated.

Q: What do you see as GAPA's main organizational problems?

A: Many of our problems are due to a lack of volunteers. Many people come in, but few stay around to carry out their responsibilities. As a result, our work just doesn't have much continuity.

Q: How has your relationship with the group been?

A: A bit difficult; maybe that's because I'm a young woman, and I don't have the same social standing as the majority of the people in the group. I think I have to fight much harder for my opinions to be taken into account. Socializing with the group is also pretty difficult. After meetings, people often decide to go to a bar or a restaurant. I would like to go with them, but I don't have the money. I'm too afraid to say so, so I make up excuses. Also, I live quite far away, and since the meetings are at night, I have to catch the last bus to get home.

Q: How many women are in GAPA right now, and what is their role?

A: There are four of us. One is a lawyer, and she takes care of all the legal business. She talks nonstop, and gives lots of public speeches. During public events or interviews, I don't have much to say about myself. When I am asked, "Who are you?" I answer, "Mônica." "And what are you doing?" Then I don't know what to say. Everyone else in GAPA has a university degree. I work in an office; that's not considered a profession. And Mônica? I am "Môniquinha" (Little Mônica), and that's it. GAPA is a group where people come and go. There is a big turnover; many people can't handle the work and leave.

Q: Have you also had problems handling it?

A: Oh, there was a period when I just had to leave. One patient, whom I had visited and whom I liked, died, and I didn't want to admit that he had died. The reality was too cruel. That's when I resolved to take a break, to think about it all.

Q: Do you have some ideas on how the group could be reorganized and how its work should be carried out?

A: I think that the group should be much more open, and that it should have a more democratic structure. But in Brazil all groups are hierarchical, so it's hard to even suggest such changes.

Q: Do you speak with your lesbian friends about your work with GAPA?

A: I talk with them, but they are not really interested. They think it's good work, but they don't want to do it. Many of them think that since they are lesbians, AIDS is not their problem. They believe that they'll never get AIDS.

Q: Do you think that your work with AIDS patients has changed you?

A: I think that the patients have taught me lots of things. I think that if I caught AIDS, I would commit suicide. Not at the beginning, as long as I could work. But later, when my life was spent going in and out of the hospital. After all I've seen, I don't think I could go through it. I don't have the financial means to be treated in a private hospital; that's way too expensive. I would have to go to the public health care system for treatment — fight for a hospital bed, receive poor care. I might even be left on a mat in the hallway — this already happened to a number of people — or even on the floor. . .

In some ways I think I've grown because of this. I think all experiences have their value, even those that are failures.

Q: Do you think that you've failed?

A: I don't know. Up until now, I've done very little. I would like to do more, but I don't have the means. If I was better off financially, I could work less, live closer to the center of town, have a car. I wouldn't become a mother to the AIDS patients, but I would be better able to help them. I would also have more time for myself. GAPA is not the reason for my existence. If I had more free time, I would also spend it doing other beautiful things with my life.

Insemination: Something More to Consider

CHERI PIES

*Cheri Pies is a health educator and reproductive rights advocate.
She is the author of* Considering Parenthood: A Workbook
for Lesbians *(Spinsters Ink, 1985).*

THOSE OF US engaged in AIDS
work often talk about the first time we heard about AIDS, in much the
same way that some people remember where they were the day John F.
Kennedy was assassinated. The first time I heard about it was in one of
my "Considering Parenting" groups in 1982. Several women raised
questions about using gay men as donors, because of this newly discovered disease and its spread in the gay male community. I have a
vague and haunting memory of not wanting to face up to the reality of
the questions. It was at that time that I began to gather all the information I could about AIDS.

I became compulsive. My files are filled with newspaper and magazine clippings from mid-1982 through 1984. I read whatever I could
find that would help me understand this disease. It slowly began to
dawn on me that I had been oblivious to the impact this disease could
have on lesbians — especially lesbians considering parenthood
through alternative fertilization, or artificial insemination.

In 1977, I started leading groups for lesbians who wanted to discuss
the many issues associated with considering parenthood. A large percentage of the women in these groups who decided to try to become
pregnant had chosen gay men as donors. I always suggested that they
get a complete and thorough medical and health history from their
donors. These medical histories were usually designed to identify
any signs of heart disease or any hereditary illnesses. Occasionally
women would ask donors about their sexual health history. They also
wanted them screened for sexually transmitted diseases prior to
donating semen.

It wasn't until sometime in 1983 that I began to suggest that lesbians
planning to use alternative fertilization techniques question their

donors more closely about past sexual activities. Even then, we had only a vague idea of what we were asking about. I did not want to discourage anyone from using gay donors. Nevertheless, we needed to be honest about what was beginning to look like a possible risk. I was acutely aware of the growing resentments in the lesbian community towards gay men and their sexual activities. I was compelled to discuss the homophobic responses of some lesbians to AIDS. At the same time, I tried to balance this discussion with a cautious warning about using donors who voluntarily reported a large number of sexual contacts. This was never easy.

Sometime in 1985, one of my professors at the Public Health School suggested I contact epidemiologist Nancy Padian, who was doing research for her doctoral dissertation at the University of California at Berkeley on the heterosexual transmission of the AIDS virus. This professor knew of my work with lesbians who were using alternative fertilization, and thought I might be able to work with Nancy on some aspects of her study. My curiosity was piqued by this idea. We met and talked about a study that would determine whether lesbians had been exposed to the AIDS virus through artificial insemination.

With the support of Nancy and Project AWARE, I began a study to determine whether lesbians who had used gay, bisexual and heterosexual men as donors had become infected with the virus through the process of insemination. We offered HIV antibody testing to any woman who had been inseminated since 1979. I thought that this study could provide a service to lesbians seeking to be tested, rather than simply be a research-oriented study.

At the beginning of the study in June 1985, there was no documentation of transmission of the AIDS virus through artificial insemination, just a hunch that it was possible, since other women were becoming infected with semen during sexual contact. A month later, a news story out of Australia reported that four heterosexual women who had been artificially inseminated at an infertility clinic in Sydney had tested positive for the virus after receiving semen from a donor found to be infected.

I never really thought that I was doing what others called "AIDS work" until someone asked me how I got involved in working in the field of AIDS. I had simply thought that providing this service and educating lesbians about insemination and exposure to the AIDS virus was all part of working with lesbians dealing with parenting issues. I have since come to realize that my contribution is very much a part of AIDS work.

So far, this study, known as the Lesbian Insemination Project or

LIP, has been one of the most challenging professional projects of my life. During the first year, I worked with three very committed volunteers who drew blood, interviewed participants, and did a variety of tasks that were essential to the project. During the second year, LIP hired three paid staff who were the backbone of the study. Because of their contribution, we could expand the project into other parts of California. Funding was provided by the University-Wide Task Force on AIDS, and other support came from volunteers and the San Francisco Women's AIDS Network.

Many lesbians who had used insemination chose not to participate in the study for various reasons. Some did not want to know if they had been exposed to the virus. Others were suspicious about the test and about whether results could really be kept anonymous and confidential. Still others were worried about their anonymity being compromised if they came to a study site and saw someone they knew. Some did not think that knowing their test result would make any difference in how they would lead their lives. There were some lesbians who knew their donors or had received semen from a local sperm bank and were able to find out the antibody status of their donor.

Of the women who participated, only half ever came back to get their test results. Many simply wanted to make a contribution to research by participating in the study. A few wanted to take the test, but later decided that they did not want to know the results. However, a handful knew that their donors were now positive. These lesbians wanted to be tested to see if they had been exposed, because there was no way to know when their donors had become infected.

Regardless of the results of this small study sample (which for funding reasons cannot yet be made public), insemination with semen from donors who are infected should be considered a high risk behavior. We know that there is a high concentration of the AIDS virus in the semen of men who are infected. When infected semen is deposited in the vagina, it is possible that infection can occur through the mucous membranes in the vagina, or through cuts, abrasions or small tears on the cervix.

All donors, regardless of sexual orientation, need to be screened for HIV antibodies at least two times prior to using their semen for insemination. Every woman using donor sperm — no matter where and from whom it is obtained — should make sure that the donor has been screened for the HIV antibody. Screening should be done twice, six months apart, before beginning insemination. If both tests are negative, and if the donor has been practicing safe sex in the meantime, this is the best assurance that the semen is uninfected. But there is no absolute certainty.

The staff of some sperm banks have suggested that women use only frozen semen. Then, after the donor has been screened over a period of six months, the woman is given the semen that was donated at the time the first HIV antibody test was taken.

I continue to remind lesbians choosing to inseminate that not all gay men are infected with the AIDS virus. This is probably the single most important piece of information I can provide. Any man could be infected, regardless of his sexual orientation. Don't assume that gay men are no longer potential donors and/or fathers. AIDS has taken an enormous toll on the gay male community, but this does not rule them out as choices for donors or partners in parenting. There are many gay men who want to be fathers, some who simply want to be donors, and others who want to explore the possibilities of co-parenting with a lesbian.

AIDS has changed a lot in this world. Sometimes I think it has changed more than we will ever know. AIDS has changed the path of the lesbian and gay parenting movement in profound ways. I grieve the loss of possibilities for parenting because of this disease, as much as I grieve the loss of friends. Somehow, though, I continue to remain hopeful that we will find ways around this threat posed to the fabric of our families.

A Selfish Kind of Giving

DEBORAH STONE

WHEN I DECIDED TO become a volunteer at the AIDS Homecare and Hospice Program in 1986, I hadn't personally experienced the AIDS-related death of someone close. However, I was aware of the devastation AIDS had inflicted on my extended community, the gay community. It took me one solid month to fill out the Hospice application form. Every day I pulled it out and read it over again. Sometimes I would write a sentence or two in answer to one of the questions, and then, defeated, I would stop. I didn't really know why I wanted to work with dying people, but I had a deep need to do something with my hands to alleviate the desperation that arose in me with each article I read about AIDS.

After I had been a volunteer for several months, I remember sitting around talking with some lesbians. The subject of AIDS came up — as it inevitably does — and I was asked about my work with Hospice. I was happy to talk about what I'd been doing. One of the women in this small group made a face. Intrigued by her look of distaste, I asked her what her reaction meant. She answered, somewhat bitterly, "Gay boys have done shit for lesbians, and now we're rushing to their bedsides. We're acting like nurses, like a bunch of mommies. Like women always do."

I carried her comment around with me for some time, mulling it over. After my initial shock at what sounded so callous when I thought of the deaths I had witnessed, I admitted that in one sense, I knew exactly what she was talking about. My response to the AIDS crisis was very much in the mold of activities considered traditional for women, not only as caregivers but as volunteers working without pay. I just hadn't heard this viewpoint stated so baldly.

Nevertheless, I couldn't see past one overwhelming fact: "People — men, gay men — are dying." So I went on sitting at the bedsides of individual men. When the opportunity to write this article came up, I used the chance to talk to other lesbians about this conflict. I was surprised that so many of the lesbians I spoke with needed very little prompting to talk about the subject. All but two of them are currently working with AIDS in some way — as volunteers, as educators, or as paid staff at an AIDS agency. Of the two lesbians I talked with who are currently not involved with AIDS, one was previously a paid staff member at Hospice; the other, a lesbian activist, prefers to commit her energies to the lesbian community.

The lives of almost all of the women I interviewed were touched by AIDS. Miriam Cantor, a bodyworker and Shanti volunteer, experienced the death of a close friend from AIDS. This was a gay man she'd become estranged from, and she didn't learn about his illness until three days before he died. She spent those last three days at his bedside. The insights gained then showed her that she could get something out of doing AIDS work and that there was a need. Shortly after, she volunteered at Shanti. "I don't feel like it was pure altruism," she said. "I knew I would get something out of it, and I have."

When I started as a Hospice volunteer, I did not know what I expected to get from doing the work, except heartache and grief. I did not think of myself as an activist, but the actions involved in doing a load of laundry, buying and putting away groceries, or providing an afternoon's relief for the immediate family of someone dying of AIDS were simple, direct and concrete. Becoming a Hospice volunteer was a way to alleviate some of my fears of death and dying and some of the hopelessness I felt about AIDS. In that sense, my work is "a very selfish giving," as one woman called her own work with the Names Project.

Each woman I talked to got something important for herself from her work. One woman, a coordinator at the Shanti Project, tells volunteers that she interviews, "We come from a selfish place, because there's something we need that we get when we do this work." Jane Halstead, who worked on the AIDS ward at San Francisco General Hospital and who is now a health care worker with the adolescent community, said many women she knows use AIDS to work out their own issues — both personally and professionally — around death and illness. In doing AIDS work, she suggested, many lesbians find alternatives to unfulfilling work. "It's a great profession in which to find your niche and to make a name for yourself," she said. "There's a sense of unity, of community. And it's a real easy thing to focus on and feel like you're doing something."

Healing Between the Gay Male and Lesbian Communities
Political and sexual differences have alienated lesbians from gay

men. Jane Halstead thinks that much of the reserve between the two communities has emanated from issues gay men have about women which they haven't yet resolved. She herself has problems with aspects of gay men's sexuality, which she sees as an extension of the "take-what-you-want, when-you-want-it, how-you-want-it, any-way-you-want-to-do-it, without-regard-for-the-consequences" male sexuality she's experienced most of her life. She observed that "gay men were so focused on creating and exploring their own culture, they just didn't want women around — just as some gay women don't want men around."

Miriam felt another kind of alienation when she began her training at Shanti. "I found much of the crowd very white, Christian and middle-class. I came home just devastated, saying, 'They'd never give me anything if it were me who needed their help. I don't know what I'm doing here.'" She realized that she was there because she expected to get something for herself. "You can't give expecting to get back," she cautioned. "Women can do all the work they want — and they are — but we're doing it for a reason, too, just like anything else."

Now, when Miriam walks into support group meetings, she still sees the same people. "But," she said, "this epidemic has really thrown them away from their identification with privilege, back to recognizing their own oppression." It has broken down barriers that kept her from relating to men in general — including many gay men. "I wouldn't have known some of these men, never in a million years — I wouldn't have wanted to go near them. Corporate executive types, with incredible homes. I come home from some of these meetings and tell my roommates — 'You wouldn't believe the way these men live!' But they're dying! It doesn't matter how they live! Sometimes I can't relate, but I always find a transcendent aspect. It's been a stretch for me. It gives me an opportunity to reach out from the heart to somebody I might not have said hello to otherwise."

For Miriam, working with AIDS clients at Shanti is an opportunity to get some of the good things men have to offer. She said, laughing, "I don't really know what those things might be, but I know that when men weren't in my life, I missed them. Giving to men and receiving from them — even though the sexual element isn't there — is really healing." Working with AIDS has been a homecoming, albeit a sad one, and a time to pay her dues. "I got something from faggots. I don't know if I'd be a lesbian if I didn't hang out with drag queens."

The greatest benefit of Miriam's work at Shanti is her exposure to people who are very different from herself. This challenges her sense of isolation and of being different. "It's amazing how much I've changed. It's not so much a me-and-them thing anymore." In learning how to reach out to people with different values, Miriam has experienced her own healing. She is not the only one. Jane Halstead also talked about healing between the lesbian and gay communities. Part of that healing has occurred because gay men have changed their priorities. "When gay men started getting sick, I felt their openness towards me increase," Jane told me. "Those changes have been based, very simply, on a survival need." Lesbians also owe a debt to gay men, according to Jane. "In the world, we are perceived as one subgroup," she said. "The boys have been fronting gayness for the girls for a long, long time. Not by choice, but because they have always been the ones who have been talked about as gay and visible."

Other women I talked to also told me that the effect of the AIDS epidemic on gay men's behavior has made it easier for them to relate to gay men. Women used to be the staid, nonsexual, verbal-therapy end of the gay community; now they see their lifestyle choices being affirmed by gay men, creating the possibility for a greater balance between the two communities. And gay men, who have felt the economic burdens caused by AIDS, may have more compassion for women, especially economically.

Despite the talk of the healing between the two communities, Miriam has doubts about how much gay men really know about the lesbian community. "From my experience in Shanti, I am not at all optimistic that gay men know anything at all about lesbians," she said. "That's a very general statement — some do — but it amazes me how much they don't want to know."

Jane Halstead no longer works within the gay community at large, which she sees as having resources for coping with AIDS. "For the most part, gay men have money, education, and choices. They have the resources they've developed within their own community and they have the resources they're getting from the lesbian community: energy, compassion, and skills." For her, this has been reason enough to extend herself outside the relatively comfortable confines of the gay community. "My approach is to take what I've learned from the gay community and move that into other areas. Shanti, Hospice and so on do not represent poor people, people of color, poor gays, or the disabled and deaf — people who don't have the ability to communicate and operate in a way that gives them access to the health care system. People who can't stand to fill out forms or who don't have addresses are not going to make it through those systems. Those systems do not acknowledge this alienation openly."

Marj Plumb, president of the board of directors of Woman, Inc., a non-residential, battered women's agency, offering a twenty-four-hour crisis line, counseling and legal support, has doubts about the "healing" or the commonality of goals between the two communities. "We're not in the same movement, no matter what we want to believe. The issues have been different since the day there were lesbians and gay men. I think it's great that lesbians are donating time and money to help, but it's wrong to think that as a result we have comrades in arms. It frustrates me that so much energy, time and money are being given under the pretense that we're all in this together and that gay men are going to react a certain way when lesbians have problems."

What Should Lesbians Expect from Gay Men?

Talking about her experiences in NOW while fundraising for the ratification of the ERA, Marj noted the absence of gay men working on that issue. Where were they when a matter of urgency faced women — and lesbians? "I don't remember seeing one gay man coming into the NOW office when we were going for the ERA. In terms of volunteer recruitment and fundraising for lesbian causes, gay men aren't around. Of course, every time you say that, you can count on someone coming up to you and saying, 'I'm a gay man and I was there.' But as a community, the response was less than enthusiastic."

I asked her if she'd seen posters for a fundraiser for the women's community produced by two women and two men and billed as the Gift Benefit. The Gift Benefit would distribute proceeds, which were originally expected to be $50,000, among eleven non-profit women's groups, including the Lesbian Rights Project, The Women's Building, Lyon-Martin Women's Health Clinic, and others. The purpose of this benefit was to show appreciation for women's efforts in the AIDS epidemic and to thank them for their work towards the "achievement of human rights for all humanity."

Marj's response was that, while she appreciated the effort, it was only a beginning. "Five thousand dollars per agency is probably a fraction of what each of those agencies needs to survive. Lesbians have very serious programs. I find it offensive that they would offer each agency less than $5,000. What do they think we're doing, recycling paper clips? And," she pointed out, laughing, "it's probably lesbians who are going to buy the tickets anyway!"

After the event, Richard Be Low, one of the organizers of the Gift Benefit, told me that they had been disappointed at the low ticket sales in the lesbian community. In the end, due to various problems, they failed to raise the targeted amount of $50,000. Asked whether he thought gay men would support the Gift Benefit's goals, he said it might be asking too much of a community that is watching friends and lovers die to support women's non-profits. Marj's response was that gay men "have to take a look at how they're feeling about things. If that is their attitude, then the lesbian community needs to start looking at their own political agendas and the things they need to be doing to survive and to flourish as a community."

These days, Marj is trying to raise funds and enlist volunteers for projects important to the lesbian community. She is frustrated to hear from women she used to be able to count on for support that all of their money — or time — has been earmarked for AIDS. The lesbian community has seen its limited financial resources siphoned off to a relatively more affluent gay men's community. At the same time, gay men have not invested time, money, or energy back into the lesbian community. "When I'm trying to get volunteers for a lesbian program, and it's more difficult every time I try, the volunteers are all going to AIDS issues and, to me, something's not right with that," Marj said.

There are a lot of issues facing the lesbian community with which gay men could help. Gay men can help lesbians open some of the doors to political and legal power. One of the most pressing things on the lesbian agenda is supporting lesbians in their bid to gain political power. Of lesbian attorney Roberta Achtenberg's campaign for the California state assembly, Marj asked, "Will the gay male community, which has more disposable income, open up their wallets and support her candidacy?"

Lesbians need to start talking to each other, Marj maintains. "I have my own emotional reactions; I've lost friends to AIDS, and I know what that feels like." Instead of a purely emotional response to the AIDS crisis, lesbians have to be able to ask hard questions as well. "This has to start in the lesbian community. We need to confront each other and ask, 'Why are you volunteering twenty hours a week for the AIDS Foundation?' Not that you shouldn't, but analyze why. When the community starts discussing these things," Marj said, "then we'll get to the reality of it."

Miriam agrees that discussion is the best route to understanding the role of the lesbian community in working with AIDS. "I don't think it takes away anything from the work that lesbians are doing to talk about this. Within that discussion, you also have to talk about what the benefits are, because if women weren't getting anything out of it, they wouldn't be doing it. But," she added, "I don't believe that just because I get all I get and bring it back to the lesbian community, that there shouldn't be some lesbian out there on the front lines saying (she pounds on the table), 'Give me money!' "

Changes in the Lesbian Community

We've all heard about the changes that have come about in the gay male community as a result of the devastation of the AIDS epidemic. Less clear are the changes in the lesbian community as a result of coping with AIDS. It wasn't until I talked to Miriam that I got a picture of what the positive aspects of the impact of AIDS on the lesbian community might be. "I think it's a universal truth that people in this society don't get to deal with grief," Miriam said. "Lesbians have a lot of grief. We're always addressing issues that bring up grief — sexuality, our children, incest and abuse histories, addictions — all of those things involve a tremendous amount of grief." Dealing with grief directly, working with it and facing it, she maintains, are activities that heal. "You can learn about how to deal with your issues through your own experience," she pointed out, "and then you can learn through others' direct experience by being in a supportive role."

She suggested that the transformational skills learned by gay women working with AIDS travel from the gay men's community back to the lesbian community. Miriam has learned about transformation by watching people accept their diagnoses and come to accept death, making living a priority. For her, this transfer takes place directly through the bodywork she does. "I see mostly women as bodywork clients, and I bring the skills I learn in Shanti to my bodywork clientele," she said. "So I bring what I've learned about transcendence and transformation back to my own community. Change can really happen," she exulted. "Change you would never believe! You look at it and say, 'Wow, look at the incredible adaptability of the human spirit!' "

I have also been transformed by people I've cared for, most especially one man whose illness kept him bedridden for the three or four months I was his volunteer. He was unable to speak, yet by the time he died I felt I knew and loved him, as much through the kind of love he received from those close to him as from an unmistakable sense of his spirit which came through. I learned from Roberto, though we never exchanged one word, that everything we use to "know" about people — speech, clothing, mannerisms, even gender — is ultimately superfluous in the face of the undeniable force of the human spirit.

Conclusion

I remember a recent phone call from a friend of mine who decided to do AIDS work and called to ask me for advice. "Volunteer at Woman, Inc.," I told her, thinking about Marj's words. She laughed. "Are you serious?" she asked, somewhat incredulous. "Yes," I said, and then summarized Marj's perspective for her. "Well, I understand that," she said, "but what I really want to do is work with AIDS." We seem to sense, every one of us, that the experience of working with AIDS will instill something lacking in our lives. Working on a phone bank for Woman, Inc., though that work needs to be done, may not satisfy those needs in the same way.

On both an individual and a community level, AIDS work, while a selfish kind of giving, has created changes for women involved in it. For some of the women I talked to, the conflicts with gay men have been resolved through the work; for others, these conflicts won't be resolved until specific actions from gay men address the economic and political inequities between the two communities. "Women are always struggling," one woman, a Hospice volunteer, told me. "It would be nice for the gay male community to get behind us and to work as one community. I mean, my god, if we had half of their support, maybe we'd be struggling half as much, too."

You Have to Know Street Talk

LEA SANCHEZ

Lea Sanchez is a co-investigator for the Lesbian AIDS Project
(LAP), which was started in July 1987. The women working for
LAP all have previous experience in AIDS outreach and educa-
tion work. The following is based on a conversation with Ines
Rieder, on January 13, 1988 in Oakland, Ca.

I'M PRESENTLY WORKING with the Lesbian AIDS Project, which is a university-funded study trying to locate lesbian IV drug users. That's not always easy; we have to go into different communities — the gay community, the drug-using community, and several ethnic communities. The Lesbian AIDS Project works on a collective basis. I get along with the other women, even though we all come from different backgrounds.

As a Latina, an ex-prostitute, and a lesbian, I'm qualified to go out into the streets and talk to people. I go to all the bars, not only lesbian bars, and just start talking with people. Sometimes it happens that I meet an IV drug-using woman in a straight bar who turns out to be a lesbian. The number of lesbians among drug users is pretty small, but still significant.

There are interesting differences that I get to observe, especially since I can pass as white if I want to. There are more white women out there who identify as lesbians, and I can pretend I am just one of them. But then when I go back to my Latina culture, it's a cultural shock every time. For white women, it's part of their culture to be out and openly public with their lesbianism. Latinas are different; we prefer to have our private parties.

When I get talking to lesbian IV drug users in the bars or on the streets, many of these women, when asked if they have sex with men, answer no. But when I ask them whether they have turned tricks, they answer yes. Look at it this way: being a prostitute is a profession. Some people might consider me bisexual since I have had sex with men for money, but I identify as a lesbian. And if you are a junkie, lesbian or not, turning tricks is often necessary to get your fixes. Even if you try whatever you can to get your money without having sex.

I think a large number of women share needles. Some of the lesbians we interviewed with the Lesbian AIDS Project share needles with gay men. It's often the same hierarchy games as in the straight world — the man takes a bigger portion, shoots up first, and then gives what is left to the woman whom he's sharing with. Once you want your fix really badly, you don't care how many people have used that needle, and you share that needle with men as well as with women. Men just have more access to these drugs, since they are the dealers. You would have trouble finding a woman who is dealing. At most, women work in the drug trade as runners.

There are two groups of drug users: the hard-core users and the weekend users. The first group comes from every walk of life. They form some kind of association with other junkies without ever being close friends. They are people from all races. I approach these hard-core drug users by telling them that I want to talk to them about AIDS. Sometimes I worry about my safety. You know, they'll do anything to get a fix; they rob, turn tricks, you name it. I carry a knife at all times for protection.

The weekend drug-using types say, "I'm a drug user, but not a junkie. I would never hustle to get drugs. I go out and work all week, and on the weekends when I have time off, I'll shoot up. I do it with anything I can get my hands on: valium, speed, crack, heroin."

I know how to talk to a lot of people from different backgrounds. There are a few Asians, but since I don't know anything about their culture, I have a hard time talking to them. I'm trying to read up on their history. If I want to educate people from other cultures, I need to find out who they are.

Since I've been in the streets talking to people, I've found that some IV drug users are highly educated people. There also seems to be a certain age limit; I would say most are between twenty-one and forty. Most of the women I've spoken to are aware of AIDS, and know something about it. I ask them if they practice safe sex. Since I was a prostitute, I know specifically what I have to ask them. You have to know street talk if you want to get anywhere.

When I started working as a prostitute, I didn't know what to say to the johns, what language to use, but I learned it pretty fast. Now I know all the key words to make these women talk. I come up to them and say, "I am not a doctor, but I know about AIDS, and this is what I think you should do." I give them condoms and tell them about using bleach for their needles. Also, I often draw their blood for the antibody test. If they come back for their results, and they have tested positive, I counsel them and help them to deal with it. I encourage them to stay in the study and receive long-term counseling from Project AWARE.

I got involved in this work through Project AWARE. When they started their study of HIV infection among prostitutes, they needed some people who would know how to talk to the girls in the streets. They thought I would be good, and asked me to do some outreach. Three of us working at Project AWARE used to be prostitutes. It's really been an experience for me. I've learned to use computers, and have overcome my fear of needles. Now I can draw blood from anyone, under almost any circumstances. Lately I've really started becoming part of the "establishment." When I worked as a prostitute, I was very private, very much in my individual world. But now I'm out there, under the eyes of the public, reaching women, and educating them on AIDS.

Five years ago I retired from prostitution and started working with COYOTE, a prostitutes' rights organization. I got involved in some outreach work to inform girls about COYOTE's rap sessions. At that time, we talked about AIDS occasionally, but it was not a big issue. I knew I had been pretty careful while working, but a couple years later, I went ahead and had myself tested. I have done three tests, and the results have always been negative.

I wanted to help prostitutes and Latinas, and now I've also added lesbians to my list of priorities. I come from a big family — we are nine brothers and sisters. They know that I was a prostitute and that I'm a lesbian. They accept me for who I am. There haven't been any big discussions or dramas about it. They all know that you have to do what you can to get money.

In order to deal with women and AIDS, we have to look at how men behave with prostitutes. There is this big difference between white men and men from minority cultures. White men are used to women who tell them that they don't want to have sex, so often you can convince them to do something else besides penetration. The guys are also already nervous, because they've lied to their wives about what they're up to — they've told their wives that they have to work overtime, or that they have a meeting to attend. With Latino men, it's different. They have told their wives, "You stay home, and I'm going out to have a good time." They are more interested in penetration; they want to put their dicks inside the women.

I guess there are some changes in sexual practices happening these days, but we've only touched the surface. Young people are becoming more aware of safe sex practices. It's important that AIDS is beginning to become part of popular culture. There are rap contests about AIDS. And there are several soap operas on the Spanish-language networks that include issues about AIDS in their plots. After all, it's hitting more and more people of color, and they have started to become involved.

I have some friends who have tested HIV positive — straight women, lesbians, gay men. Some of them have used drugs. Some I've known for a long time. Some I met through my work. Once they find out that they are positive, they say that they want to be celibate. I always tell them, "Don't deprive yourself." In the end, very few stay away from sex. They just have to get over the hurdle of being positive.

V

Prostitution in the Age of AIDS

EVEN THOUGH THE specifics of the transmission of HIV, especially heterosexual transmission to men, are still among the many gray areas of AIDS research, prostitutes have been singled out as the group responsible for passing the virus to straight men, and in turn to their unsuspecting female partners. Warnings to stay away from prostitutes are an international phenomenon.

In Asian countries where prostitution is a major component of the tourism industry, such as Thailand and the Philippines, few AIDS cases have been reported so far. Clearly, these governments, which profit from the influx of foreign exchange by tourists and military personnel enjoying the night life, may not be motivated to report accurately about infection rates among sex workers. Women's organizations in the Philippines and Thailand have also begun their own educational campaigns. Empower, an organization for sex workers in Bangkok, Thailand has distributed posters in toilets of hotels and bars, reminding women to use condoms.

The Caribbean and Central America have also seen rising numbers of HIV infection, due to North American sex tourism and marines in search of a war. On some Caribbean islands, large numbers of male and female prostitutes have been infected, while in countries with a strong foreign military presence, like Honduras, infection seems to be mostly among women who serve GIs.

In many African countries, prostitutes are blamed for the spread of AIDS in the large urban centers. Some reports claim that large numbers of these women are HIV-positive. However, it remains unclear how systematic the data collection has been. In some countries, concerned women have begun to involve prostitutes in AIDS education projects. In Nairobi, Kenya, for example, prostitutes have been invited to participate in community health workshops since January 1985. Safer sex methods are discussed, and a year after the first workshop, half of all the women who had attended were insisting that their customers use condoms all the time, and the other half most of the time.

In the United States and throughout Europe, infection rates among sex workers who do not use IV drugs have been very low. Surveys in West Germany, for example, found that less than one percent of the registered prostitutes are HIV-positive. Studies in the United States have also shown that HIV infection rates among professional sex workers are insignificant. Infection rates among IV drug-using prostitutes — in Europe as well as the United States — are much higher. Many of these women not only engage in risky needle-sharing practices, but are also often willing to provide unsafe sexual services. In contrast, those women who consider prostitution as a regular profession are very concerned with their health and take all possible precautions to protect themselves and their customers from infection.

Hookers with AIDS—The Search

LYNN HAMPTON

CRUISING DOWN THAT stretch of Peachtree Street the hippies used to call The Strip, past the taco place, past the old drugstore, down by the Krystal, you'll see them: the remains of the street people. Here are the burnt-out druggies, the winos, the shake-down artists, the pimps and their ladies.

I'm standing on the corner watching a young white hooker change her blouse in a parked car in the Krystal parking lot and wondering whether she's incredibly defiant or just stupid. Everybody knows whores aren't allowed in the Krystal lot. Rumor has it that the fat white rent-a-cop who keeps the women out of the joint shot a black hooker in the spine for mouthing off when he told her to haul her freight. Could be true.

Now the woman gets out of the car and strolls across the lot in my direction. She doesn't look like she's afraid she'll be blown away any minute, and she doesn't look particularly defiant, either. I decide she just doesn't know what she's doing, and I call out, "Hey, mama. What's happening?"

She glances at me with little but disinterest. I'm obviously not a trick, and she doesn't make me for a police woman, either, so whoever I am, I can't be that important. "Not too much," she replies.

I fish in my green canvas shoulder bag and pull out a handful of prophylactics. "Can you use some of these?"

Now she registers some interest. "Sure. Thanks." She's looking at me with vague suspicion, wondering what's the catch.

"It's not real healthy for working girls to be on the Krystal property," I tell her. "And the rent-a-cop gets pretty weird, I've heard." I smile to let her know I'm one of the good guys.

"Oh, wow. Thanks."

I pull out one of my cards and hand it to her. The logo is a woman in a corset wearing fishnet stockings. Underneath, it says, "I'm for

H.I.R.E.," and under that, "Hooking is Real Employment." In the bottom left corner is my name, "Sunny" Lynn Hampton, Vice President. We're a prostitute's rights advocacy group in Atlanta, with the decriminalization of prostitution as our goal.

"Far out," she says, and pokes the card into her back pocket.

"I'm the one putting up all these posters about free AIDS testing. You seen 'em?" I ask.

"Yeah. What's the story?"

"Well, the Feds are trying to find out if working girls are carrying the AIDS virus. So far, it doesn't look that way, at least in Atlanta. I've tested about sixty women and nobody's got it so far. Anyway, it's a good chance to get tested, for free and anonymously. We're also testing for hepatitis B and syphilis. Wanna do it?"

"Gee, I don't know, man. How does it work?"

"I ask you a bunch of questions and fill out a questionnaire. Then I draw a tube of blood. That's it. Takes about half an hour."

"I don't know. . .You won't put my name on anything?"

"No. Just a number. Come on. I'll give you more rubbers."

"Okay," she shrugs. I interview her over a beer in the taco place and bleed her in the john.

This job and I were made for each other. The Department of Human Resources lucked out when they found me. What they needed was someone who could establish credibility with the women, someone comfortable with street people, not some tight-assed social worker or nurse with a white coat and a bad attitude. They also needed someone who could draw blood samples, somebody mighty good at it, too, who could tap blood even in a junkie whose veins were long since shot.

When I heard about it, I jumped at the chance, already knowing the job was mine. I was an advocate for hooker's rights, I had ten years of experience as a medical technician, and I knew the street scene from my days as a flower child in the late '60s. Who could ask for more? And the money was great.

I found that nothing had changed much on the streets in the years since bell bottoms and peace signs disappeared. Same dirty streets, same sleazy joints, same drugs, just new faces buying and selling them.

It took a week or so for people to get used to seeing me around, drinking beer in the joints, talking to people, giving condoms to the working girls.

Then I met Sam.

"Ain't you the rubber lady?" she asked.

"Is that what they're calling me?" I laughed. "Yeah, that's me. You need some rubbers?"

"Shoot, yeah. Gimme a bunch."

I gave her a handful of condoms. "You know, I'm not just the good fairy of condoms," I said, "I need some interviews from you ladies, too. Make my day. C'mon. I'll give you more rubbers after the interview."

Later, her blood sample safe in its styrofoam sheath in my bag, we chatted over a beer while she waited for her man, Poochie, to come. She was eager to explain that Poochie was her boyfriend, not her pimp.

"What's the difference?" I wanted to know.

"Well, a pimp says he loves you and makes you work and beats you up if you don't. But Poochie, he really loves me. We been together four years. He don't make me work. I'm just doin' this until he can find a job. He don't hardly ever hit me, either," she beamed.

Sam was white, said she was twenty-seven, but looked thirty-five. I guess it had been a long, hard road.

Suddenly a young black man entered the taco joint and approached us. "You got any money?" he asked Sam.

"Hey, baby! Yeah, I got $80." She handed him a wad of bills. "This here is the rubber lady. She gave me an AIDS test and a whole bunch of rubbers."

He nodded at me. "That's good."

One day I stood in front of the topless bar across the street from the Krystal watching a young black hooker plying her trade. I was just about to approach her when Poochie walked up behind me. "What's happenin', man?" he said.

"Say, Pooch. Not too much. I was just fixing to hit on that hooker over there." He looked at the woman, then at me and grinned. "I don't think I'd bother," he said. "She ain't no 'ho. She a boy."

"C'mon, man. You kidding me?"

"Nah, I ain't kiddin'. She a 'ho, but she a boy, too. You just doin' real women, right?"

"Yeah. Damn." The woman crossed the street toward me. Sure enough. The Adam's apple always gives them away.

Jennifer was the name she gave me. She was twenty-three, blonde and pretty, despite her thinness and the black eye. On the inside of her elbows were bruises ranging from last week's brown to today's deep purple, the unmistakable tracks of a heavy cocaine shooter. She was bright, with a caustic, quick wit and flashing smile. I liked her. "C'mon, Jennifer," I said after the interview, "You've got to start using condoms. If you don't, it's just a matter of time. And your needles. Do you share needles?"

"Honey, when I buy them, sometimes they're at right angles."

"You're not serious."

"Hell yes, I'm serious. What do you think, I just walk into a drugstore and say, 'Excuse me, sir. May I have some sterile points, please? And a half pound of pharmaceutical cocaine, while you're at it?' Shit, I'm lucky to get needles at all. And you're telling me I may get a disease that will kill me five years from now? Honey, I'm amazed I'm alive right now. If I'm alive two weeks from now, I'll be doubly amazed. I've got to come up with $400 each and every day, just to put in my arm. That doesn't include rent, food and trips to Rome, honey. Just to feed my veins. That's what I have to worry about, not some disease that may kill me in five years. Get real."

Sometimes I worked with a partner. One of them was David, a bright young sociologist. David was gay, and rather small in stature. We were working Ponce de Leon Avenue one night, even sleazier and more dangerous than The Strip, when suddenly, behind us we heard, "You! Wait! Wait for Sherry!"

We stopped and turned to look. Running toward us as fast as her size thirteen pumps could carry her was the ugliest transvestite I'd ever seen: Six-foot-four, about 220 pounds, waving her arms frantically with a look of utter terror on her painted face. She was done up in a blue satin dress, size eighteen at least, with a feather boa flapping behind in her wake. In the dim light of a street lamp, I saw a nasty razor scar from cheekbone to nostril that no amount of makeup could hide.

"Oh, thank God!" she cried, winded and panting. "There's a car full of rednecks after me. Can I walk with you as far as the Starvin' Marvin to call a cab? I'm afraid they'll get me."

David reached up to pat her shoulder. "Calm down," he said. "We'll take care of you."

And the three of us strolled down that funky, dirty old street, the huge scar-faced black man in a blue dress and feather boa protected by a fat middle-aged woman and a small gay man.

Sometimes you have to laugh.

We went to a halfway house to give a safe sex talk and interview the women. These were women halfway out of prison — not quite in jail, not quite ready for the street. Most of them were in for drug-related offenses, and there's no such thing as a female drug addict who doesn't turn tricks. We got eighteen blood samples that day.

Most of the women were black; a third were white. One of them was twenty-three and had been in prison for four years. Her veins were fine — no scar tissue at all. "You in for a drug offense?" I asked, bending over her arm.

"No."

I untied the tourniquet, looking up. "What, then?"

"Murder. I killed my husband."

I was stunned for a moment. "Well, I hope he needed killing," I said. Her blue eyes didn't waver. "He did," she replied.

Plum Nellie's is a funny kind of a bar. An old woman, with hands twisted from rheumatoid arthritis, plays the piano while gay boys sing Broadway show tunes, camp it up and flirt. In the back, pimps in snakeskin boots and leather coats wait for their ladies.

I'd been waiting, too. Six or seven rum-and-Cokes had made the wait easier, and I was drunk enough to not be aware how truly strange a spectacle I made in the place. The gay boys ignored me; the pimps glanced at me with amused looks and shrugged to each other while I smiled benignly at everyone.

It was 1:00 a.m. and still no whores.

"That's one helluva hunk of gold you got there," I said to a young pimp standing next to me. He detached himself from his friends to glance my way, fingering the gold chain around his neck. The thing must have weighed half a pound.

"Yeah," he said.

"Business must be pretty good," I slurred.

"Not too bad," he replied, his eyes suspicious.

"That's good. That's good. Too bad it won't stay that way." I let my voice trail off.

"What you talkin' about?"

"Well, I've been doing the free AIDS tests for working girls. Maybe you've seen my posters. Anyway, most of them aren't using rubbers regularly."

"So what?" He was vaguely hostile.

"They're all gonna die, man. It's just a matter of time." I sipped my drink, giving him time to digest what I'd said.

It didn't take long.

"But these women ain't fuckin' no faggots. How they gonna get AIDS?"

"Because they're running drugs with other people's points, man. And they're fucking bisexuals. Like I said, it's just a matter of time."

"No shit. Say, why don't you gimme some rubbers? I'm gonna make my chicks use 'em."

I dug into the green bag for condoms.

"What else you got in that bag?"

"Oh, I've got my blood tubes, needles, interview forms, stuff like that. Why?"

He looked at me for a long moment. "You're pretty drunk, ain't ya?"

I thought about it for a second. Everything was kind of fuzzy. "Yeah, I am a wee bit stinko, now that you mention it."

"Why don't you let me call you a cab? There's people around here who'd take you off in a heartbeat just for them needles."

I blinked. "Take me off. You mean . . . off? Oh, wow."

I let him call a cab.

Only about 20 percent of prostitutes are streetwalkers. The other 80 percent are call girls and escort agency workers. In order to make our study representative of the entire spectrum of working women, I needed an equal number of these women. To find them, I advertised in a local newspaper.

One of the women who responded was a forty-five-year-old named Cindy. Cindy ran a massage parlor out of her apartment and not only worked herself, but employed five or six other women, too.

Cindy was a woman with a goal. She had lived in India for twelve years and had put together a project to build model villages there for orphans. She intended to go back to India in some comfort, however, and decided that she needed $40,000 to live in style while organizing her orphan village. She had amassed $30,000 in nine months.

Here's to free enterprise and the American way.

Late one night, I interviewed two women, using the dim light of a neon sign in a window to read the questions on my questionnaire. I wasn't too sure about these ladies. They were too well dressed.

One was very attractive and wore a clingy black dress short enough to reveal her very shapely legs; the other was tall and slender, blond and very fair of skin. Her prettiness was spoiled by severe acne scars. She wore tight leather jeans and a lavender halter which defined her bosom. Their makeup was impeccable.

This was early on in the study, and I hadn't yet realized that the women who work Peachtree Street don't look like the stereotypical whore. If you see a woman with a short dress and fishnet stockings with high heels, you can bet she's either a cop or a boy. The RG's (real girls) wear bluejeans and T-shirts. They don't carry purses, many wear no makeup and inevitably they wear sneakers.

You can't run in high heels.

The two were cooperative and honest. I read the questions about numbers of partners, about drug use. No problem. When I got to the section about birth control, I asked what types they had used in the past five years. They each replied that they used condoms occasionally. No birth control pills. No IUD's, no diaphragms.

"How many times have you been pregnant?"

"None."

The light began to dawn. I already knew what the answer to my next question would be.

"How old were you when you started having your periods?"

They glanced at each other nervously. "Uh . . . I don't know. . . Like, thirteen."

"Uh, yeah, about thirteen. Me too."

Right. What could I do? Embarrass them? Say something like, "Gee, ladies, this survey is for RG's only?" Or, "Wow, you really had me fooled! Gosh, what they can do with silicone these days!"

Besides, if they were living as women, working as women, and were in the process of becoming women through surgery and hormones, what the hell was the difference? I finished the interview, drew their blood, gave them condoms and wished them well.

Next day, in the office of the Department of Human Resources, I explained to Terry what had happened.

"You got two blood samples from a couple of transsexuals?"

"Yeah, I did. What can I say. And they were gorgeous, man."

"Well," she thought for a moment. "We'll submit the samples with an explanation. That way, they can still get their results."

The Department and the Centers for Disease Control decided not use the interviews as part of the data for the study, so even though I drew 125 blood samples all together, 123 was the official count.

The study lasted from February 1986 to February 1987. Of 123 blood samples, one was positive for HIV antibodies. She was a drug addict from Florida, who shared needles. She had never turned a trick in the state of Georgia.

The other cities testing prostitutes had similar results, proving what some of us already knew — prostitutes don't have AIDS, junkies do. Every hooker infected with HIV is a drug user first and foremost, who uses prostitution to support her drug habit, and she got it from an infected needle.

An article in the October 24, 1986 *Journal of the American Medical Association* states, "Since infection is transmitted to only about 10 to 50 percent of steady heterosexual partners, the likelihood of transmission to a partner with a single exposure must be quite low, *probably less than 1 percent per contact.*" (Italics mine.)

With this being true, it's unlikely that a prostitute could infect a client even without the use of a condom, and there is little chance if a condom is used. Still, month by month, toward the end of the study, the numbers of women working Peachtree Street and Ponce de Leon decreased as police sweeps "cleaned up" the area of "disease-ridden" prostitutes.

The Georgia Department of Human Resources, even with only one HIV-positive blood sample from 123 working women, still recommended the mandatory testing of all convicted prostitutes. As a taxpayer, I kind of resent that.

Toward the end of the study, David and I walked the circle from Peachtree to Tenth Street to Juniper and back many times on a Saturday night without seeing a single whore working the street. I guess you could say Atlanta has conquered the "prostitute problem." The street whores of Midtown have been harassed and arrested right out of existence.

To me, it's a little embarrassing. A city as cosmopolitan and sophisticated as Atlanta claims to be with no hookers on Peachtree? New York has 42nd Street. San Francisco has the Tenderloin. Baltimore has The Block, but there's no mo' 'ho's on Peachtree no mo', y'all.

If a city's sophistication can be judged in part by its view on sexuality, what shall we say about Atlanta? What was it Mammy said to Rhett? "You can put a mule in a race-horse harness, but it still ain't nothin' but a mule."

Poochie and Sam are gone now. Sherry no longer clatters down Ponce in her size thirteen pumps. Jennifer is gone. Plum Nellie's is gone, too. Even Cindy is gone, off to India to build her orphan village.

I guess it's a good thing. The young upwardly mobile couples who rushed to midtown to buy up the fine old houses while they were still cheap can breathe a sigh of relief. Fancy hotels and condos and office high-rises have changed the face of Midtown, and the Strip is now the cultural center.

That's progress.

Still, the hookers took a little of the old flavor and color of Atlanta with them when they went away. . .Oh, well. Git up, mule.

Occupational Hazards

PEARLIE, CHERBY AND PONG

In Olongapo, a city in the Philippines adjacent to the U.S. naval base of Subic Bay, the booming "hospitality" business employs about 15,000 women. They work in bars, massage parlors and restaurants catering to U.S. servicemen on "rest and recreation." Although hospitality workers receive very low pay, their salaries are often higher than those of maids, waitresses or shop clerks. And, in any case, employment opportunities in such fields are very limited. Prostitution has also become a major component of the tourist industry in the Philippines.

BUKLOD (a Tagolog word meaning bond) is a community center for hospitality workers in Olongapo, established in cooperation with GABRIELA, an umbrella organization for many autonomous women's groups and projects. Anju Gurnani, an acupuncturist interested in women's health issues, visited BUKLOD to find out how AIDS has affected the lives of these hospitality workers. She spoke with Cherby, a hospitality worker; Pearlie, who used to work in the hospitality industry, but is now a community worker at the center; and Pong, a community organizer who helped establish BUKLOD. During this conversation, "having AIDS" refers to those who have tested positive for the HIV antibody; no distinction is made between those who have AIDS-related symptoms and those who are HIV-positive without symptoms.

Q: Can you tell me something about your work at BUKLOD?
Pong: BUKLOD was started in 1987. Hospitality workers come to BUKLOD to chat, rest or drink coffee. We also give workshops on a variety of topics. We just finished one on contraception and abortion. We discuss women's identity and women's rights.
Pearlie: I came to the center because I liked the idea of self-sufficiency, and because they offer English lessons. Now I have become a full-time community worker with BUKLOD. This is much better than working in the bars. I talk to the girls in the bars as a friend. I ask them to come here and attend workshops.
Q: Has the working situation here changed because of AIDS?

Cherby: It hasn't changed much. But we have to be much more careful. Before it was just syphilis and gonorrhea; there are just too many diseases now.

Q: What kind of medical treatment is available for women who get sick with syphilis or gonorrhea?

Cherby: One of my friends got VD. The Social Hygiene [a government-run health center for Olongapo's hospitality girls] gave her medicine. When she went back, she had VD again! She decided to go to a private clinic instead, but that is just too expensive.

Pearlie: Every time the women make love, they take antibiotics. They just buy them in the drugstores. A lot of women don't even use contraceptives. They think that the antibiotics will keep them from getting pregnant.

Q: Has the government taken a role in educating hospitality workers about AIDS?

Cherby: We had our first workshop about AIDS last week, sponsored by Social Hygiene. They were supposed to show us a slide show about AIDS, but the projector broke. They explained how we can take care of ourselves with customers. They told us to use a rubber when we have contact with somebody, in order to avoid AIDS, and to wash everything with warm water and soap after every contact.

Pearlie: In Olongapo, twenty-four girls and one gay man have AIDS. All of the women are still working in the bars. The test results are confidential and we don't get to see them. I guess that Social Hygiene just doesn't know what to do for the girls, so they don't tell them.

Q: How were the tests carried out?

Cherby: Last month, they told us to go to the Social Hygiene to get an AIDS test. They came to the bars and talked to our managers, who told us to go. We've all gotten the test. Last year was the first time we took it. And now we've had the second test. Every year we pay 200 pesos (about U.S. $10) for medical examinations, which include the AIDS tests. We also have to pay a little extra for each blood smear for gonorrhea, which we have twice a month.

Q: Have you always used rubbers, or is this something new?

Cherby: Before, most of us didn't use rubbers, but now we use them more. Social Hygiene gives us the rubbers.

Q: How do the customers react to using condoms?

Cherby: I don't do that kind of work much any more. I just go once in a while, with my old customers. I told one man to use a rubber, and he agreed, even though he said it's better not to use it. I told him that I was worried about getting pregnant. I didn't mention the disease. Some customers say they aren't satisfied with the rubber.

Q: Is there any conflict with the Catholic church because condom use is promoted?

Pong: The church is not such a problem. It is not so much against condom use, but it is adamantly against abortion. The real difficulty is the customers; they don't like using condoms. Of course, if a woman needs money, she'll go ahead and have sex without the condoms. And if she won't, the customer will complain to the bar manager and the woman will get in trouble.

Q: Is there anything working women can do, given that their work is controlled by bar managers?

Pong: We are trying to educate the managers and build a relationship with them. Some of the managers are women — female pimps. It's not easy to deal with them. One of them did want to join our center. We accepted her as a member, and now she is helping us.

Q: You mentioned before that twenty-four women have tested HIV-positive, and that they are still working. . . .

Pearlie: Yes. How can they support their families and pay the rent unless they work? The Social Hygiene knows that they are infected. They should put them in a hospital or do something.

Cherby: I've heard that Social Hygiene tells the bar managers who has AIDS. They tell them not to let the customers pay bar fines for those infected. [A customer pays the manager a bar fine to take a girl out. Usually some sexual service is expected.] But girls will still go out with guys; they can negotiate on their own.

Pearlie: Maybe the government is afraid that if they tell us who has AIDS, the infected women will just commit suicide. They wouldn't be able to work anymore, or support their families. They may also be afraid that the girls will ask the government for assistance.

Q: Do many of the women here take drugs?

Cherby: Yes, most do. If they are under the drug, they won't be shy. I think many girls take Valium, speed and marijuana. I haven't heard of women using injections.

Pearlie: Women take drugs in order to feel more comfortable dancing naked and all of that.

Q: What about the military base? Are they involved in educating people about AIDS around here?

Cherby: The U.S. base supports the Social Hygiene, providing medicines for VD and rubbers. If the base closed, Social Hygiene wouldn't be there. I think all of the instruments they use for tests come from the base.

Pong: It's like paying for damages.

Cherby: I talked about this to one marine, who said that the captain

167

gives condoms to all of the marines, every day, when they are having morning formation. Sometimes they just make balloons out of them, or throw them away.

Pearlie: Very few of the guys take this seriously, or will use condoms. They have educational workshops before their stay at the base here. They are warned about getting VD and are told not to take too much money with them once they go off the base. It's all to protect the guys. They protect the servicemen, but not the working women.

Cherby: If they know that a girl has AIDS, they pass that information around on the base. I've heard that there are pictures of all of the girls posted inside the base. If a girl has AIDS, they turn her picture upside down. Also, if certain bars are known to have a lot of VD, they are avoided by the servicemen.

Q: What are GABRIELA's plans regarding future AIDS prevention among hospitality workers?

Pong: GABRIELA and other organizations are demanding that all foreigners coming into the Philippines must have AIDS tests. We've also demanded that if women get AIDS, the government must support them for life. Filipinas have to work as prostitutes because of basic economic problems, and if they catch this virus, what will happen to their families?

GABRIELA is working together with HAIN (Health Alert Information Network), a non-governmental organization of medical professionals, trying to do research and education regarding AIDS. They have produced some informational brochures on AIDS for the hospitality workers. They are researching different diseases, like AIDS, and how their rates of infection correlate with other STDs.

We plan to start our own clinic soon. Hopefully every weekend some volunteers will come here to help. We want to monitor the health situation of the hospitality workers. And we want to include people who know about AIDS testing. The problem is funding. Right now we can only refer women to other doctors who will offer their services at low cost or free. But we can't afford to buy medicine or testing supplies.

We can't wait for the government to take care of the AIDS problem among the hospitality workers. The government is not thinking about how big this problem could get.

A Chronology, of Sorts

PRISCILLA ALEXANDER

*Priscilla Alexander is co-director of COYOTE, a prostitutes'
rights organization, and education coordinator of CAL-PEP. She
co-edited* Sex Work: Writings by Women in the Sex Industry *(Cleis Press, 1987).*

FROM THE FIRST time I read
about this strange new disease in August 1981 while working for a
medical society in San Francisco, I became engaged in the quest. Sorting out the mail, I looked at all the medical journals carrying articles
about a disease that seemed to exclusively affect gay men. When sexual transmission was brought up as one of the possible causes, I knew
that sooner or later women would be drawn into it, since sexually
transmitted diseases had never ever singled out one sex or the other.
Because of my many years of involvement in the fight for prostitutes'
rights, I figured that prostitutes would, in some way, become involved
in this new mystery.

By the spring of 1983, AIDS began to pose serious problems for lesbians, gay men, bisexuals, and other sexually stigmatized groups, by
setting the stage for major civil rights violations. As a result, I worked
on a resolution for a regional NOW conference which supported
NOW chapters' involvement in promoting AIDS research and support services for AIDS patients, while opposing any moves to limit the
civil and human rights of lesbians, gay men, bisexuals and others.

At the first National Hookers Convention in San Francisco, organized in 1984 by COYOTE, we discussed the possibility that, by changing their sex practices, prostitutes could be leading the fight against
AIDS — if this new disease was, in fact, sexually transmitted. At that
time most street prostitutes used condoms fairly regularly — at least
on the job — while off-street prostitutes were less likely to do so.

Although no tests had been done to show whether condoms blocked
the transmission of the virus, condoms are effective in preventing the
passing of other sexually transmitted diseases. At the convention, lots
of time was spent talking about how to use condoms properly. Using a
cucumber, one experienced prostitute demonstrated how to put a

condom on a customer with her mouth, without the customer ever knowing it had been done.

By late 1984, medical "authorities" talked more and more about the possibility that prostitutes could spread AIDS to the heterosexual population. But no one ever expressed concern that prostitutes might get the disease from their customers. We stepped up our promotion of condom use, and we discussed it with every prostitute in our network.

Project AWARE began its study of women presumed to be at risk for AIDS in April 1985. Women were defined as being at risk if they had had either five or more male sex partners in the previous three years, or one or more male sex partners with known risk behavior. The study has included prostitutes. It was the first, and, as of this writing, the only study of any significant scale to directly compare prostitutes and non-prostitutes for risk of infection.

Meanwhile, in Seattle, the Director of Public Health had begun forcibly testing women who had been arrested for prostitution. Using the highly fallible ELISA test, he found that 4.5 percent of them were infected. This figure was widely publicized and was used as documentation for those wishing to blame prostitutes for the spread of AIDS. We learned much later that these women were re-tested with the more accurate Western Blot test, and they all were negative. But the Seattle director has yet to publish this fact.

It was in the summer of 1985, after the report from Seattle and a similar report from a small study at an AIDS screening clinic in Miami, that the scapegoating of prostitutes for the heterosexual spread of the AIDS virus began full force. At the second National Hookers Convention, we discussed AIDS at great length and developed statements and policies on mandatory testing, quarantines, pregnancy, risk reduction measures and the need for public education. At that time, condoms were never mentioned on television and rarely in print, although their efficacy in preventing the spread of AIDS was known. We also discussed the common police practice of confiscating or damaging condoms when arresting prostitutes.

The condom had its television debut in the fall of 1985 when representatives from COYOTE, including myself, appeared on a segment of the "Today" show, discussing the importance of using condoms to prevent AIDS. The station's switchboard lit up, and Bryant Gumbel apologized for our controversial discussion.

By late 1985, results from various studies of prostitutes were in. The more significant and informative results came from the Project AWARE study, which included a control group of heterosexually active non-prostitutes. Much to everyone's surprise, except our own, the incidence of infection, 4.5 percent, was the same in both groups. However, the more startling fact was that, among the prostitutes, all of those infected were women with a personal history of IV drug use, so that their probable means of infection was shared needles, while prostitutes not using IV drugs tested negative. A major difference between the prostitute and non-prostitute group was that condom use was much higher among the prostitutes.

Project AWARE's study was one of seven funded by the CDC. Most of the other studies looked only at prostitutes, without a control group, and used an extremely skewed population of prostitutes — often those most likely to be using IV drugs. For example, they tested women at jail, at sexually transmitted disease clinics and in methadone maintenance programs. Only two studies, the one in San Francisco and the one in Atlanta, looked at a broad range of prostitutes.

Despite the deficiencies in these studies, the results substantiated those in San Francisco — that infection was directly related to either a personal history of IV drug use or an ongoing relationship with an IV drug user. One study of brothel prostitutes in Nevada found none to be infected. The highest incidence of infection was in New Jersey, where women were tested in a methadone program. The CDC reported that the incidence of infection among prostitutes mirrored that of all women in a geographic area, and that IV drug use, not prostitution, appeared to be the deciding factor determining infection.

After the CDC issued its report, the media's scapegoating of prostitutes declined somewhat, but much damage had already been done. Many states have introduced legislation for the mandatory testing of prostitutes. Georgia, Florida, Utah and Nevada now forcibly test at least some prostitutes, and at this writing California is considering a similar law. And in several states, district attorneys have attempted to charge some prostitutes with attempted murder or attempted manslaughter, because they have continued to work although infected. In Orlando, Fla., a woman was charged with manslaughter even though she used a condom with all her clients, and all of her clients who had been tested came out negative.

In 1987, COYOTE was approached by the AIDS Activity Office of the California Department of Health, and was asked to submit a proposal for an AIDS prevention project for prostitutes. As a result, the California Prostitutes Education Project (CAL-PEP) was formed to do educational service projects from an office near one of San Francisco's stroll districts. Outreach workers, all of whom had worked as prostitutes, meet with prostitutes to discuss safe sex practices, distribute condoms and bleach bottles, and invite them to a weekly support group to discuss means to reduce the risk of AIDS infection.

Later that year, due to pressure by COYOTE, the Department of Health and others, San Francisco's police department became the first to issue a special order prohibiting the police from confiscating condoms or bleach from suspects.

We have been contacted by public health departments and AIDS projects around the country requesting information on how to develop AIDS prevention projects. The first thing we say is that the most important element to a successful program is to hire prostitutes to develop and staff the project and, surprisingly, most agree to this. And so, perhaps for the first time in history, experience as a prostitute is becoming a requirement for legitimate employment.

Gloria Lockett and I had our second appearance on the Today Show in January 1988. Gloria Steinem was presenting a segment on our AIDS prevention program. This time, two and a half years later, we not only talked about condoms, but we also showed a variety of condom packages on the air. Bryant Gumbel was, again, the host, but this time he felt no need to apologize. So things are changing.

However, recently, in an otherwise excellent AIDS information program distributed by HBO, Surgeon General C. Everett Koop spent the requisite one hour talking realistically about sex and stressing abstinence and monogamy as a way to reduce the risk. But he admitted that not all people could adhere to that, and so he advised the use of condoms.

When he talked about prostitutes, he accurately explained that some prostitutes who were IV drug users were infected with AIDS and that they continue to work in order to pay for their drugs. However, instead of saying that customers should use condoms as a result, his final comment on the subject was, "Don't have sex with prostitutes." I mean, business is down, but there are still a lot of men hiring prostitutes, and he knows that. So why was he unable to give realistic advice, as he did concerning other sexual contexts? Through this program he had exhorted the audience to have compassion for gay men, but when it came to prostitutes he lacked that same sympathy.

As this battle rages on, be alert to the scapegoating that goes on, and fight it. We must not stand by while stigmatized groups — female or male — are blamed. Because, in the end, it doesn't only damage specific groups, but all of us.

Dominating the Crisis

MISTRESS MORGAN

I AM A THIRTY-TWO-year-old woman living in Atlanta and working on my B.A. in journalism at Georgia State University. I am a lesbian feminist witch, joyfully creating my life in the New Age. I write a column for our gay center's newspaper, and for the last nine years I have earned my living as an outlaw sex worker. The AIDS epidemic has changed the way I work and live.

I began working as a call girl in 1979, when the only consequence of sex I worried about was pregnancy, and an IUD took care of that. However, I was concerned about my health and appearance — I took vitamins, ate well, exercised and got my rest. In short, I cared for my immune system because I did not want to get sick and miss work.

When I first began hooking, I fully engaged in sex with my clients. I kissed and frenched them, touched their bodies with my hands and tongue, performed fellatio and intercourse without a condom, and I allowed them to touch me and perform cunnilingus. I had sex while menstruating, but I wore a diaphragm to hold back my menses. I also provided domination services, which are theatrical fantasy sessions of bondage, humiliation, discipline and costuming and which often included giving my clients anal intercourse with my bare hand or a condom-covered dildo. Nonetheless, I never induced rectal bleeding.

I always washed a client's genitals before sex and inspected them for signs of disease or parasites. I would refuse service to any suspicious person. I also followed other common sense hygiene practices, such as not passing germs from the anus to the vagina and rinsing my mouth out after sex. In addition, I thoroughly washed myself before and after each encounter.

About five years ago, the media's messages about AIDS began sinking into my brain. It was hard to believe that sex could kill you, but I heeded the warnings and began haphazardly using condoms during intercourse and fellatio. I say haphazardly because sometimes I felt too intimidated to insist on their use, or they slipped off inside me, or I just couldn't bear the taste of any more latex. I would make a client wear one for intercourse, but not for fellatio. Sometimes, my clients asked me if I was worried about AIDS, and I would say I was being careful. But in truth, I was only hoping and praying that my number would not come up.

Sure, I was worried, but I rationalized that most of my clients were married and had few sex partners and were not sleeping with men or using needles — I thought the risk was reduced. Yet, I was troubled about the times I had whored in the Caribbean, because Haitians were considered a high risk group then and I didn't know if I had ever had sex with one. When I found out that the other two hookers I had worked with at that time had not contracted AIDS, I figured I probably hadn't either. I did not get tested because I was afraid of being told I would die. But when I got too freaked out about it, I stopped seeing clients for weeks or months at a time. My lesbian lovers supported me when I got the Hooker Blues, but I missed whoring and devised a plan to work safely.

Two years ago, I made the decision to become a full-time dominatrix and give up genital sex work. I believed that this form of prostitution would gain in popularity as the public became more aware of AIDS and afraid of multi-partner genital sex. Domination games do not include genital sex; in fact, most times the Mistress remains totally dressed while the submissive is naked or dressed in a kinky costume. The client's orgasm is self-produced, or the Mistress may masturbate him while wearing latex gloves. Domination is safe sex, and my clients appreciated my commitment to stopping the spread of the disease.

One year ago, I attended my first safe sex party. Our university's Gay Student Alliance sponsored the event. I tearfully came out as a prostitute and shared my fear about getting tested. I wasn't going to pass it on if I had it, because of my new domination work, but I was terrified of being tested. I was not pressured to get tested, and if I chose to do it, I would do it anonymously.

It disturbed me to know that women could contract the disease through cunnilingus or from contact with menstrual blood. Information about women's or lesbians' risky sex practices was rarely included in articles about AIDS. This news frightened my lover, and she wanted me to get tested right away. We stopped having oral sex, but the worrying about AIDS chipped away at our relationship, so that we separated six months ago.

Finally, after breaking off with my lover, I got tested. I wanted to have sex with a new lover, who insisted that I be tested. She is an AIDS educator and a prostitute and had tested negative. She gave me the courage to do it, and even went with me for the results two weeks after the sample was drawn.

As I waited for the results, I was an emotional wreck. I insisted that if it was positive I would sell my house, quit school, and travel around the world. I planned to kill myself as soon as I got sick. If I had the virus, I was determined to live my last years as fast and furious as I possibly could. But I never intended to infect anyone, and I was committed to telling future sex partners that I was a carrier.

I was thrilled to learn that my results were negative.

If we all assume that everyone else has the virus, and we practice safe sex, AIDS can become a disease of choice and can be avoided. Furthermore, AIDS is everyone's concern, and we all can help fight the disease. I take part in a bimonthly healing circle that welcomes people with AIDS and other diseases. We meditate, visualize, and pray for the healing of the sick. And we ask for continuing strength to the healers and speedy discovery of a cure by the researchers. We heal each other through touch. Mostly, we open our hearts and allow the universal energy, which some call god, to work through us and make us compassionate and loving people. The AIDS epidemic has its challenges, but it also has its gifts. My wish is that all people allow their spiritual selves to emerge and heal themselves.

VI

Becoming Visible: Women AIDS Educators

INCREASINGLY, AIDS HAS become a focus of women's professional lives, even for those in fields not traditionally associated with the epidemic. Many have found themselves researching, reporting or organizing on the AIDS front.

Professional involvement and volunteer labor by women was instrumental in building the infrastructures of the many educational, material and emotional support systems available today. Particularly in the United States, AIDS education and organizing is dependent on grassroots efforts, due to the minimal response and support by the federal government. In most other countries, governments, often together with gay activists, have taken on the educational and financial responsibility of dealing with AIDS-related issues.

Obviously, bureaucracies alone are not sufficient in dealing with such a demanding task. Crises demand the dedication and skills of people who are willing to give more than their forty-hour work week. Although the amount of labor by women staff and volunteers in AIDS organizations is difficult to assess, it is obvious by walking into any of these organizations that women's work is an essential component of their structures.

Despite the large number of women doing AIDS work, their participation is not often publicly visible. Many AIDS organizations are either run by men or strictly under men's control. The male organizers are the ones who are known and are quoted in the papers. Their voices are heard on the radio, and their faces appear on television.

Many women AIDS activists have responded to this invisibility by creating their own networks, in both the United States and Western Europe. These autonomous networks allow women from all AIDS-related fields to come together to discuss issues that are relevant to their current work, as well as plan projects and propose policy recommendations regarding AIDS issues of specific concern to women. As the number of women with AIDS and those working in AIDS organizations grows, these networks alone may not be enough, and the established hierarchies will have to accommodate more women.

For Many a Long Month

RUTH SCHWARTZ

Ruth Schwartz is Educational Events Coordinator of the San Francisco AIDS Foundation, and an active member of the Women's AIDS Network.

October 1980

CHARLIE AND I hunch over our poems, the jug of pink wine on the table between us. Brian waits at the door, impatient. It's 3:00 a.m.; I want to stay up with Charlie, talking about his men and mine, his poems and mine. Brian, whom Charlie calls "Butch" because of his cocky walk, wants me with him.

Charlie is there the night Brian spies on me from the roof, the night Brian puts his hand through the glass. Brian is a hemophiliac, so it is no small thing when his fist comes through the window. I bandage Brian, but Charlie's sympathies are with me, my restlessness. He, too, has broken free from lovers; we unite in our refusal to be tamed.

Charlie is brilliant, irreverent; he makes fun of the men whose hearts I am breaking, the men who are breaking my heart. Some nights, he is half carried home, drunk, from parties at which he wanted to get laid, and didn't. Other nights, I marvel at the way he moves, fluidly, between all the men who are his lovers and friends. It's the same way he moves through the kitchen, gracefully bursting the cloves of garlic with the knife's brown arm, twirling to stir the soup.

January 1986

The San Francisco AIDS Foundation's office manager welcomes me, shows me around. Here is the supply closet: paper, envelopes, an oxygen tank. Here are the lounge, the bathroom, and the hotline area, where people hunch over telephones, saying things like, "When you're giving a blow job, don't let him come in your mouth," and "Yes, your cock has to be hard before you can put it on." Here are the boxes of condoms, the stacks of T-shirts emblazoned "Bartenders Against AIDS."

Something tells me this job will be unlike any other job.

My mother is horrified. "You're committing suicide. Nobody really knows how AIDS is spread. You're going to get it and die. Couldn't you work somewhere else, like the American Cancer Society? Why choose to walk right into a job that might kill you?" My lover and friends are curious, but supportive. They don't know much about AIDS, but they figure it would be fun to work around a lot of gay people.

But when I talk to Brian, he tells me that he is infected with the AIDS virus. His health is fine, but of course he has no way of knowing when he became infected. Most hemophiliacs in the United States received AIDS-contaminated blood products between 1981 and 1983. Brian and I were lovers until July 1982.

My lover is frightened. I tell her, "Even if I were infected, we'd be making medical history if I infected you. There are no reported cases of women infecting other women through sex." Actually, doctors have already seen a case of woman-to-woman transmission, but it will be nearly a year before it makes its way into the medical literature.

February 1986

My mother is visiting. She doesn't want to see where I work; she is still fearful. I say nastily, "Mother, if I were going to get AIDS, that's not how I would get it. Remember Brian, whom you liked so much?"

Still, not knowing is different from knowing. Now my mother knows there's a possibility I could be infected, but that's a thousand times removed from a reality. When I contemplate taking the test, I think: if I test positive, she will be afraid to see me.

I decide to get tested through Project AWARE, a study researching women at sexual risk for AIDS. They define such women as "women who have had more than five sexual partners in the past three years, or women who have had a partner they know to be infected." I qualify under the latter category, though I have been in a monogamous lesbian relationship for over three years.

Before the blood test, I answer a lengthy oral questionnaire about my sexual practices. It seems that Brian and I had a lot of very high-risk sex.

I am shaking as we finish the questionnaire. It's time for the interviewer to draw my blood. I've had blood drawn before, but this time I feel terrified of the needle. She tries for a vein, misses. She apologizes; it's the end of a long day for her. She calls in someone else. The second woman hits my vein on the first try, fills two test tubes with my blood. Then I am free to go.

It will be two weeks before I can get my results. While waiting, I learn that another old girlfriend of Brian's — one who came after me — was also tested through Project AWARE, but decided not to go back for her results. I can't imagine making such a choice. But then, I work at the AIDS Foundation; every day I am surrounded by AIDS. What will my relationship to this disease be? I have to know.

I remember Charlie, moving gracefully through his affairs. We were roommates in the winter of 1980, the spring of 1981. Now I know that during those months, doctors in Los Angeles and New York were seeing the first cases of a new, mysterious immune deficiency in gay men.

March 1986

My test results are negative. I feel relieved, but also guilty. Many of the men I work with are infected. Several have ARC. One was recently diagnosed with AIDS. My risk was real, but it is over now, and I am safe. Their risk continues.

I brush my teeth and my gums bleed. I think about how it would feel to know that that blood could kill someone.

Charlie and I lost touch years ago; after college, it seemed he entered a gay male enclave which had no room for me. Now I realize I entered my own enclave too: Brian, security, our fantasies of the future together. Since I came out as a lesbian, I've wished I could tell Charlie; I want him to approve.

Now, in the Foundation's waiting room, I am seeing men who look like him. I surreptitiously approach each one — hoping it will be him, hoping more that it won't be.

May 1986

I join the Women's AIDS Network, a volunteer group which provides information, support, and advocacy on women's AIDS concerns. I am on the committee which authors the first AIDS brochure to target lesbians, "Lesbians and AIDS: What's the Connection?" We discuss lesbian risk and safe sex, and include a section describing other ways in which lesbians are affected by AIDS: socially, emotionally, psychologically.

Soon, we are receiving requests for the brochure from all over the United States, all over the world. We've barely publicized it, but somehow word got out; lesbians are increasingly eager, even desperate, for the information.

Meanwhile, at the AIDS Foundation, "Women and AIDS" is the most requested pamphlet; over 150,000 copies will be distributed this year. Does this huge demand for material reflect a corresponding change in behavior? Are women taking steps to protect themselves? No one knows.

November 1986

At a weekend training, I meet Meredith — the first woman with

AIDS I've actually spoken to. I am startled because her last name is Jewish, because her style of dress is like that of my friends.

Meredith has just moved from New York. She is full of horror stories about the hundreds of women with AIDS there: women isolated in one hospital with their babies in another, women refusing medical treatment for themselves in order to be with their children, women isolating themselves from each other because of their fear, guilt, shame. Meredith is grateful for the support she's received from gay men, but, she says, it has its limits. "It's hard when I'm in a group of PWAs (people with AIDS) trying to talk about my vaginal infections, and I know half the guys have never even seen a vagina, and the other half are thinking 'yuck'. . ."

December 1986

The Annals of Internal Medicine prints a letter reporting "an apparent case of woman-to-woman transmission of HIV," commonly known as the virus which causes AIDS. Now, lesbian safe sex has become more than a theoretical issue.

January 1987

I have been reading about hairy leukoplakia, a fungus that creates thick, velvety-looking patches on the tongue, common in people with AIDS and ARC. In the bathroom at work, I examine my tongue. It has a strange, thick coating on it. It looks like it's covered with little, whitish hairs. If it's not hairy leukoplakia, maybe it's thrush, another infection common among people with AIDS. I tell myself it's nothing, go back to my desk, try to work. I can't concentrate. I go back to the bathroom, look at my tongue some more. I think: What if my test results were wrong? What if they mixed my blood up with someone else's?

Finally, I approach a nurse who is working at the Foundation. "Pat, I know this is going to sound ridiculous, but. . .I was just looking at my tongue, and. . .it looks sort of funny. . .would you mind taking a look at it?"

To her credit, she doesn't laugh. She looks at my tongue, says it looks normal to her. Still, I don't really believe her until I get home, with people I'm comfortable with. One by one, I get all my housemates to stick out their tongues. They all look the same as mine. It's just that I had never looked so closely at tongues before.

Eric, a childhood friend of Charlie's, calls me, hoping I'll know where Charlie is. I'd been hoping he would know.

March 1987

At the Fifth National AIDS Forum (which is also the National Lesbian/Gay Health Conference) in Los Angeles, I sit by the Sheraton Hotel pool, marveling at how far we dykes and faggots have come. I also begin to wonder whether we have come in the right direction. The AIDS Foundation has almost doubled in size in the fourteen months I've been there; it has become increasingly slick, "professional." Evidently, we're not alone; this conference radiates the same professionalism. The expertise is real, but there is also an arrogance which disturbs me.

On a personal level, it feels good; I enjoy making a decent salary and working at an agency that has earned worldwide respect. At the same time, I wonder what the Foundation loses as it moves further and further from a grassroots, community-based effort.

Most of us around the pool are white, middle-class, gay men and lesbians, while the U.S. AIDS epidemic is striking more and more poor, heterosexual people of color. Will we be able to take AIDS work where it needs to go — or even to let go enough to let others take it there?

May 1987

On vacation in Mexico, I dream about Charlie. I want badly to be in touch with him. My lover suggests that I put a personal ad in one of the gay male papers; there's bound to be someone in the city who knows him. I make plans to do this.

But when I get back to the city, a letter from Eric is waiting for me: "I got a call from Charlie a couple of weeks ago — during a seder, actually — and he was calling to let me know he has AIDS. It was so great to hear his voice, and so awful to hear the news."

June 1987

In a letter to a friend, I write, "It was eerie when I talked to Charlie tonight — he's living in New Orleans now, but he'd just gotten back from San Francisco yesterday. He came out here to set things up, as he's moving back here for treatment and support, and he was at the AIDS Foundation office just last week. I didn't see him there, but I easily could have.

"Despite my work at the Foundation for a year and a half, AIDS has still felt somehow distant from my life. All the people with AIDS that I've known have been people I met through work; I think that's allowed me to pretend that the disease is localized, that people I've known in other contexts, times and places are not getting sick. News of Charlie's illness feels like a blow in the stomach. It's *real*. . .

"I remember feeling shell-shocked for a while, when I first began having more contact with women with AIDS. But after a while I got used to it, and was able to distance myself from 'those' women, and see them as different from the women I knew in the rest of my life.

"But Charlie feels like such a part of my past, my life. It hurts so much, feels so unfair. And understanding the enormity of the context in which he is dying makes it so much more infuriating, devastating. Another one of the thousands upon thousands of faggots dying.

"I feel bad for writing about him like this — as if I am eulogizing him when he isn't yet dead. I hope I will be able to be with him, be close to him. But I am angry, too, because I wanted things from him: his perspective on me as I used to be and how I've changed; his sharp wit; his part of the meager sense of continuity in my life."

July 1987

"Straight people are so fucked-up," Charlie used to say, and I'd laugh, hearing it not as judgment but as observation. I remind him of this when I come out to him. "Gay people are fucked-up, too," he tells me wearily. "Of course — but I hope at least I'm less fucked-up as a gay person than I was as a straight person," I say. That gets a laugh out of him, and we make a date for dinner for the following week. "I promise not to die before next week," he says, "but I'm not making any promises for the week after that."

He had pneumocystis in March, and now he is going blind. We are in a Japanese restaurant, and I pour his tea. Still elegant, he swirls it like a fine wine, tastes it, pronounces it too light, pours it back into the pot. Moments later, pouring my own tea, I hear the chorus of AIDS hotline workers in my head: the virus must get directly into the blood stream to infect; the concentration of virus in saliva is so low that it would take a quart of saliva to infect; the virus is fragile, dies in hot water. Yet I feel the fear beneath my thin layer of knowledge, even as I raise my teacup to my lips.

Charlie reaches for his cup and almost knocks it over. CMV (cyto-megalovirus) has already blinded one of his eyes; now it is slashing through the other, red with burst blood vessels. His conversation is the same — tales of museums in Berlin, culture in Italy, food in France, poverty and night life in Brazil — but his body is an old man's, gaunt and wizened. Then he tells me about the attack he had last week, when he was suddenly unable to move. It was as if the commands going from his brain to his limbs just didn't work. Now he's afraid to be alone, in case it happens again.

This isn't Charlie, not the Charlie I want. Back at his house, he can't find the copy of the Berkeley journal that published his poems; he says he doesn't feel like writing any more.

August 1987

At work, I ask people about Charlie's medical conditions, get answers about treatments and prognoses, but there is no room for grief. We are educators with a lot of work to do, and our work doesn't encompass emotion.

I attend a lesbian birthday party decorated in "Early Dental Dam"; dozens of the little latex squares are draped delicately from streamers, hung in graceful arches over the doors. There is controversy in the community about this; some vigorously promote dental dams as the women's equivalent of condoms, while others believe oral sex is safe, especially between women.

Every lesbian friend has a question for me. "Three years ago, I slept with a man who shot up in front of me. At the time, I was trying to be cool. What are the chances that I got exposed?" "Last year, I slept with a woman who used to use IV drugs. I know she shared needles with a lot of gay men. When we had sex, I bled a little. Should I take the test?" "An old boyfriend of mine was bisexual. Lately, I've had sore throats all the time. Do you think I should be worried?"

Most lesbians whom I know have some conceivable AIDS risk in their past or present lives; however, for the vast majority, the risk is very slight. At times their anxiety irks me, just as I am sometimes irked by the AIDS hotline's heterosexual callers, people panicked because of one-night stands they had years ago. Their fear seems self-indulgent compared to the concerns of people who are actually at risk, or infected, or have ARC or AIDS. Compared to Charlie, for instance.

Still, I know everyone's concerns are valid. After all, as our speaker's bureau says, "Everyone needs to know enough about AIDS to know whether or not they're at risk, and to evaluate the behavior changes they may need to make." Besides, I've had my share of irrational fears.

September 1987

Charlie is dead. "I don't need to ask what from," says Brian, limping downhill from his house above the Castro. No, he doesn't need to ask what from.

Brian has no AIDS-related symptoms, but the joint problems related to his hemophilia have worsened — partly because of the period of time before the blood supply was screened, when avoiding transfusions was his only protection.

I remember the plans we'd made when I was sixteen, the children we were going to have — a red-haired daughter first. When Factor VIII concentrate was developed in 1964, Brian was seven years old; he became part of the first generation of hemophiliacs who could expect to have a normal lifespan. Now, all that has changed.

When I'd told Charlie that Brian was infected, he'd said, "That makes me so angry — people who didn't even get to have the fun, getting the disease." But I didn't want Charlie to believe his fun had brought on his disease. Now, I want anger from Brian, not disquiet resignation.

October 1987

One of the women with AIDS who has been most active — giving speeches, being interviewed on radio and TV — has had another bout of pneumocystis; now she is homebound. The Women's AIDS Network chips in to buy her a VCR.

I get a phone call from Catholic Charities. Another woman, a client of theirs and ours, has a son in Los Angeles who's just had a nervous breakdown. The son's doctors think it will help him to see his mother; part of his panic is about her illness. She has no money to fly down there, and she is too sick to take the bus. Can we help with the plane fare?

Another woman client's daughter recently died of an overdose. She needs money for a dress to wear to the funeral.

And these are just the luxury needs, the "extras." There is still no San Francisco housing program for women with AIDS who have dependent children, or women who want to live with their partners. The AIDS Foundation food bank provides no extra food allotments for women with children. Few drug treatment programs will admit women who are infected, much less women who have ARC or AIDS; many women seeking drug treatment are placed on waiting lists.

Meanwhile, the Women's AIDS Network continues to receive telephone and written requests for information from women all over the world. We do what we can, and the AIDS Foundation helps, but we have no funding or staff to answer this onslaught of requests.

November 1987

At the Lesbian Agenda for Action Conference, I speak at a workshop on "Lesbians and the Politics of AIDS." In my remarks I try to make a woman with AIDS come alive for the group. I describe her: how she ignores her symptoms for months, caring for her family; how she is finally diagnosed after the diagnosis of both her boyfriend and her baby; how she is sterilized against her will when she goes for an abortion; how few services are available to her.

I discuss the question of lesbian AIDS risk. Contracting AIDS will never be a huge problem for women who have sex only with other women and who don't use IV drugs; but AIDS forces us lesbians to examine our political allegiances. The civil rights struggles of people of color and of gay men are also ours. AIDS also connects us to the women's health movement with its teachings about preventive health care and to sex industry workers, many of whom are lesbians, who are being scapegoated, but not always educated, about AIDS.

After the speakers, the group launches into a heated debate. Many women are concerned at the "disproportionate" amount of attention AIDS receives in the lesbian community; after all, far more women die of breast cancer every year. Others fear that lesbians are cementing themselves into an all too familiar caretaking role through our involvement with AIDS work.

Finally the moderator calls on a woman who's had her hand up for at least ten minutes. "I am a lesbian, a woman of color, and a mother. I am also a former IV drug user, and I was married to a man who died from using. No one can tell me that AIDS isn't my issue," she says simply.

December 1987

Services for people with AIDS are plentiful in San Francisco, but even here, resources are slim for women with AIDS, particularly women with children. In San Francisco, 98 percent of AIDS cases are still among gay and bisexual men. Though many of us fear these statistics will be very different in a few years, right now the bulk of services are targeted toward gay men, and the lion's share of the too-small AIDS resource pie goes to gay white men. Many of us have begun to say the words "gay white men" quickly, slurring them into one word, "gaywhitemen," seeing them as the privileged, the powermongers of the epidemic. There is some truth in this. Yet now when I say "gaywhitemen," I think of Charlie's face, the ruby flecks piercing his eye, his skin shrinking into his bones.

Communities Under Siege

SUNNY RUMSEY

Sunny Rumsey is the coordinator of the AIDS Outreach Pro-
grams at the New York City Department of Health. The Depart-
ment's AIDS Unit was started in February 1985, and Sunny was
one of the original staff members. At first, the AIDS Unit
operated a hotline to provide information and counseling for the
HIV antibody test. The AIDS Unit grew from employing fifteen
people to a staff of more than fifty counselors and outreach
workers. Now Sunny trains representatives from community and
health organizations in New York, as well as across the country,
to provide AIDS education in their specific communities and
professional settings. Sunny comes from a family of organizers ac-
tive in the black Caribbean community. The following is based on
an interview with Ines Rieder in New York City on June 2, 1988.

IN 1975 THE MINORITY com-
munities were very tense because they were afraid. People of color
weren't getting any education, and gay men of color were also often
missed, because they are in the closet and they don't identify with the
gay organizations. They are gay when they're in the Village, but when
they go home to their grandmothers and sit down for chicken and
rice, everybody is straight. They just "happened" to be living by themselves for the last twenty years. Gay people of color know that their
community is also their support system, and to come out of the closet
means taking a chance. They might be ostracized from that community, and then where would they go? The gay white community isn't em-
bracing them.

If you tell the average person that there are about 4,000 men of
color at risk, most people will assume that 80 to 90 percent are drug
users, and maybe 10 percent are gay or bisexual. In reality, almost half
of these men are gay or bi. That's something these communities are
not dealing with. And even those men who admit to bisexual behavior
are still considered straight by their communities.

This is a big problem for minority women. Take professional black
women, for example. They go out with these men, thinking that they
are not at risk. They believe that they can tell who is gay or bi. In

minority communities, these things are still perceived in a stereotypical way. You tell them about the risks, and they say, "Of course I won't have sex with an IV drug user or a gay man. The guy I'm dating makes sixty thou; he's an accountant." They believe that they'll be able to tell who'll put them at risk, and they often guess wrong.

They believe if they are married, they are not at risk. They believe if they are white, they are not at risk. They believe that if they have a certain income level, they are not at risk. And they believe if he is doing something, he'll come and tell them. With poor women it's the same. Their men are their support system. Most IV drug-using men do not tell their women that they are taking drugs, and women have no way of knowing. We have to teach these women the concept of empowerment, so they can control the situation.

For example, we hope to make it possible for a woman who has been infected by her husband, who died two years ago, to stay in the community rather than being thrown out. The city doesn't have an apartment for her, or a condo in Florida. If her community doesn't accept her, chances are good she'll end up in the streets. She'll live in the subway, infected, with two kids in tow, or in a shelter, which is just as grisly. And who'll help her with her kids when she gets sick? Nobody. And we don't have a single program set up for these women.

I think here in New York we are pretty realistic about these issues. We tell people around the country not to look at us as Sodom and Gomorrah, but to look at our blueprints. Take us as an example of what you'll have to do in your community. Avoid our constant crisis, where we don't have time to play catch-up. By the time we talked about infected women, we already had infected babies.

People react with anger and resentment and lots of denial. The media has portrayed this as a gay white male disease, which is only now hitting the minority communities. But long before the media attention, people in our communities had been saying that this was genocide. Why? Because their experience of AIDS is one of benign neglect. Or, they suspect the government of specifically putting a virus out into this population to eliminate it.

New York is one of the eight states that still has a law on the books that says if you carry needles, you can be arrested. This sets up the behavior for sharing them. In the late 1960s, the black movement was raising all kinds of hell, and then the black community was flooded with heroin, to break the back of the black movement. You flood them with heroin, you set them up to do the needles, and then you make a law that says they have to share them. And on top of it, you have a virus that's transmitted sexually and by blood.

Our society has to look at what we want to do with that virus. What's the level of compassion in this country? Remember how the house of the white family in Florida with the three hemophiliac sons was burnt down? You know what the minority community folks said: "Shit, if they treat the white folks like that, you know they are goin' to do it to us." How can I respond to that? Show them examples of where they have been treated better?

We tell them that regardless of genocide, regardless of their feelings — which we understand — it doesn't change transmission: the virus is sexually transmitted.

Many kids across the country ask me, "If I gave X a blow job, and if I had anal intercourse with Y, can I still get pregnant?" Or, "I heard that I am sterile until I'm eighteen." And another kid told me that he is Catholic and can't use condoms, but that he's using Glad bags instead. Kids are sexually active, just like adults. They are in a culture that's sex-obsessed.

We remind parents, "Don't teach your kids to say no; half of them already said yes!" When we meet a mother who tells her daughter to say no — but doesn't want anyone to tell her about AIDS — we let her know that she's putting her grandchild up on the line.

There is no sex education in the Caribbean community, but then many communities are like that. You don't talk sex with your family, let alone a stranger. It's impolite.

There is an illusion in society at large that we are setting up outreach programs for minority women. If you look at the programs across the country, what do they do? They offer fifteen minutes of counseling and a condom. It might take a woman seven sessions to discuss what to do, let alone decide whether to start carrying condoms. But there are no allowances for that.

Government officials think that the minority communities are just waiting. But minority communities are defining AIDS policy for themselves. You can give them all the literature you want, but until men of color understand why they must use condoms to save women's lives, you aren't going to see a bunch of women of color standing up in their community. What would they do? Fight their men? Walk away with their kids? Will they say, "I'm going to assert myself, I'll leave and go grow up."? Go where? Are you going to take her in? Do we have halfway houses for women of color across the country? What are their realities?

In the Caribbean community, as in most third world communities, the male is still the symbolic head of the household. Even if society doesn't recognize him, and even if women live off public assistance, many women of color continue to go to the authority of the male for the final say.

AIDS has just highlighted a lot of problems which already existed. The minority community knew about these problems, but the gay community wasn't bothered by them before. Now, when they are trying to access the system, they are raising hell. And the minorities are saying, "Welcome to the deal."

We can't let ourselves get depressed, though. We understand clearly the overall goal. And if we don't do everything we can now, shame on us. In ten years nobody will need AIDS outreach. Even in five years they won't need it. They'll need social services. You'll have a population that will be so sick, everybody will have to take care of them, whether they like it or not.

I have to face my ancestors. How can I face them if I don't do everything I can to try to save my people? How can I look myself in the mirror if I don't do what I'm doing? There are people who started AIDS work because they had listened to my lectures. Or, after sitting with them for five hours, they start doing AIDS outreach work. You can't look at it as just a job; you have to realize that you are out there — not just to save people of color, but *people.*

The City of New York now has a five-year plan, and it looks pretty good on paper. But that five-year plan should have been here five years earlier. We are reacting and not preparing, and there's a big difference. Our national policy is to say no, to be cautious, to be monogamous — to go back to the good old days. But there are no government plans for the future. There is no emphasis on giving minorities money to study social work. The people who want to study for their business degrees get support, but how will that teach people to take care of someone with AIDS?

There are no rewards for being a social worker. There is no money for social services. It's something that must come out from the heart. And how does that come from the heart when we have been raised in a narcissistic culture? This is the Me Generation. The generation that sees the differences among us, and not how we are the same. For the AIDS virus, that's not a luxury that the earth can afford. If we don't understand how AIDS affects us as women, regardless of where we live, we will lose the battle. Because if one woman loses, we all lose.

Caution Rather Than Panic

ERIKA PARSA

*By April 1988, West Germany had 1,973 reported cases of people
with AIDS, among them 112 women and 10 girls.*

I STARTED WORKING with the
Berliner Aids-Hilfe (AIDS Assistance) at the beginning of 1987. I was
the first person hired to deal specifically with AIDS issues for women
and children. At that time the organization had just realized the need
to have someone specializing in this area.

Originally the Aids-Hilfe office was located in four small rooms in
an apartment building right next to a freeway. The whole house
vibrated from the traffic whizzing by. Three phones rang nonstop;
lots of people were coming and going. I often felt as if I worked in a
congested railroad station. The workload was overwhelming; most of
my colleagues were close to nervous breakdowns. I thought I had
entered total chaos. Recently we moved to a comfortable downtown
office. There is still too much work, but our surroundings are more
comfortable now.

Aids-Hilfe Women's Group

My first contact with a woman client is when she comes for an HIV
antibody test. The counseling session usually lasts one to two hours.
However, when one of my clients receives a positive test result, I often
spend more time going over options and encouraging her to get further help and to join a support group.

So far, only a few women who have tested positive have been willing
to join a group to talk about themselves. The majority of the women
are devastated and have remained isolated. One woman told me, "For
one and a half years, I hoped that I would wake up in the morning and
this nightmare would be over. They would tell me that the results were
wrong. I took the test three times to confirm the results. I was extremely lonely until I joined this group."

The Aids-Hilfe offers self-help groups for gay men, former junkies,
relatives of people with AIDS, and, since April 1987, women. In the
women's group we talk about all aspects of this threatening infec-

191

tion — how to tell one's friends, family and acquaintances, how to deal with a new partner. The group allows women to talk about death, dying, sexuality.

Women who are HIV-positive have many specific concerns. For instance, there are women whose babies' antibody status is still unclear. In most cases they are single mothers in rather desperate circumstances, without emotional or social support. The majority of infected women with children have a history of drug use, and many are still using. Some hope that with the birth of a baby everything will change. This often remains a dream, and they end up more isolated and lonely than before.

These women need a special support system which allows them to have some time to themselves. As a result, a government-funded support group for mothers was started. It is not a self-help group, but is organized by a social worker. Each of the women in the group receives assistance taking care of legal, medical and practical problems, as well as child care.

Our group has established contacts with other women's groups, in order to carry out joint actions to respond to AIDS issues involving women. For example, the city of Berlin wanted to routinely test women who had been raped for the HIV antibody, whether or not they'd requested such a test. We believe that women who have been raped should be tested only if they've given their consent and if the appropriate counseling is available. Women's organizations have worked together to protest this action. We also follow and protest cases of discrimination due to AIDS.

Fidelity — A Political Issue

Fidelity is portrayed by the government as the only safety in the midst of the AIDS epidemic. The West German government sponsored a film spot — to be shown on TV and in movie theaters — which admonished us all: "Be careful if you are sexually intimate with changing partners! Each new partner increases your risk for AIDS. Avoid risky encounters; fidelity is the best protection!"

If you follow this reasoning, you can conclude that you have to stick to one partner, simply because both of you have tested negative for the AIDS antibodies. This puts a lot of pressure on relationships. It creates uncertainty, which can exacerbate existing problems for relationships already suffering from poor communication and mistrust. The fidelity solution to the AIDS epidemic acts almost as a threat, coercing couples to stay together.

Safe sex recommendations are based on the use of condoms. This brings up many questions. Does this mean that we all have to use condoms, under all circumstances, for the rest of our lives? I am sure that this is neither necessary nor realistic. Who has to use them, when and for how long? Does the beginning or the continuation of a relationship depend on the condom?

Suggesting the use of condoms during the first sexual intercourse with a partner could create distrust and provoke fearful and jealous fantasies about a partner's present and past sexual life. I can also imagine people becoming afraid, suspicious and abusive when a condom isn't used.

Use of condoms has declined in recent years, with large numbers of women taking the birth control pill. The pill has allowed women to experience their sexuality more freely without fear of pregnancy. The image of the sexually independent, autonomous woman is very popular these days. But in many cases this "liberation" is superficial. For instance, few women question the assumption that they must take all responsibility for birth control. In fact, this burden has somehow become equated with woman's sexual freedom. Now, because AIDS prevention requires men to wear condoms, many women are questioning their previously selfless behavior.

Nowadays there is plenty of AIDS information throughout West Germany. But this education is only meaningful if people are willing to act accordingly. Both partners have to take responsibility if they want to have risk-free sexual contact. Women will have to learn to insist on the use of a condom, even if her partner resists. Safe sex requires that both partners modify their sexual behavior within the context of their relationships.

A Report From the Front Lines

LAURIE GARRETT

*Laurie Garrett, currently a biomedical correspondent for News-
day, and a former science reporter for National Public Radio,
has covered AIDS issues since August 1981.*

OVER THE YEARS, I have worked
in research hospitals and covered countless medical stories. But I still
can't get used to seeing a child, desperately ill, crying in pain. Last
year, the AIDS epidemic took me to Children's Hospital in Newark. I
met a five-year-old boy whose chest heaved regularly in heavy bouts of
coughing. He was in the outpatient clinic, getting his weekly checkup
and gamma globulin shots: injections his doctors hoped would help
him fight off AIDS. His coughing betrayed a bad bout of pneumonia
— a common problem for children with AIDS. His teen-age mother
tried to comfort him, stroking his hair and kissing his sweating brow,
but he howled loudly between coughing fits, "Please, Mommy, please!
Don't make me get a shot." She promised him a movie if he behaved,
but the boy was not up for bribery.

What she couldn't make the child understand was that the pain he
was experiencing at the moment was his only miniscule hope for a few
more weeks of life. She said she had passed the AIDS virus to her son
during pregnancy. But, she hastily added, she got the virus from the
boy's father, a junkie who, as she put it, "Is a no-good lowlife who I
hope is dead."

Such raw and bitter emotions are difficult to absorb. I grew up in a
white, middle-class suburb, attended "all the right schools," and
studied science. I'm not street tough. But AIDS has forced me, and my
colleagues, to come to grips with realities many Americans generally
try not to think about. As the epidemic spread into our country's
toughest ghettos it brought me to neighborhoods the cops don't dare
patrol anymore. In Newark, I walked through the bombed-out rubble
and abandoned buildings that are holdovers from the city's 1967 race
riots, past preteen boys who openly carried guns and sneered,
"What's a white bitch doing here?"

I met most of the street people of Newark through Gregory Howard. For ten years Howard roamed the streets of Newark in search of heroin. When I met Gregory Howard, he was on methadone treatment, worked as an AIDS counselor for a local substance abuse clinic and was single-handedly raising his adopted four-year-old son. Howard approached his daily work with almost missionary zeal, grabbing junkies off the streets and telling them about AIDS. The more time I spent with Gregory Howard, the more I identified with him. We are the same age, enjoy the same music, laugh at the same jokes, and both love extra-rare juicy hamburgers with everything on them.

But Gregory Howard's life couldn't have been more different from mine. He grew up in the ghetto and started shooting heroin during high school. He has obvious scars that attest to years of street life, and he has always lived in poverty. As we drove down the Newark streets, Howard would point to buildings in states of abominable disrepair and say, "Now that one, that ain't half bad. I wouldn't mind at all getting myself and my son into that building. He wouldn't see no people shooting heroin in the lobby of that one." I found that the only way Newark's AIDS crisis could be viewed was through the eyes of a person like Gregory Howard.

We talked to a woman in Howard's old neighborhood. Betty went to high school with Howard, and, he said, "always seemed like one of the ones who might make it out of here." Now Betty was strung out on heroin, weaving back and forth, dressed in skin-tight alluring clothing, monitored at all times by her sullen, silent pimp. Howard tried to convince Betty to check into the methadone clinic and get a free AIDS test. He gave her a government coupon good for twelve weeks of methadone and an AIDS test. I asked her if she planned to use the coupon.

"Yes," she said, "AIDS is first and foremost why I'm going to do it. Because you never think about it until it's on your doorstep. And it's on my doorstep, since I know a couple of people that the Lord has taken in this manner. So, I mean, it's just like anything else. I don't want to wait, you know? As of now I'm free of any type of disease, even a cold. And I want to keep it that way. I have just recently got tested, in November. And that was voluntary. And not just AIDS, an entire physical."

I didn't quite believe her, and asked again, "They say you're not infected?"

"No. And I just had a baby last year, and the baby is drug-free. I was drug-free at the time. But the baby was premature and all she had to do was gain weight. No disease, no infections. So I feel the Lord has been very good to me, considering the type of life I have led. I have been pushing my luck. Lord, just give me a couple more days until I get to this clinic and you know I'll be all right. I'm not pushing it anymore."

"I hope you make it," I said.

"Thank you," she replied. And then shyly she asked if she could hear what she sounded like on my tape recorder. I hesitated, and shot a glance at Howard. He nodded, with a sad look on his face. I rolled the tape back a few minutes, turned up the playback volume, and let Betty hear herself. A raspy, low, slurred voice rambled in free association, sometimes coherent, but often completely incomprehensible.

After Betty listened for a couple of minutes, tears rolled down her cheeks, and her whole face fell. She gasped and said, "I didn't know I sounded that bad." I turned off the tape recorder and glanced again at Howard, asking with my eyes for a way out of this one. He turned to Betty and asked quickly about a few old high school chums, chatted about his parents, and then said his good-byes.

Howard and I walked a few blocks before either of us said a word. Howard finally broke the silence. "It really amazes me, but I guess that's how I looked and how I was. And to have come so far and gotten myself together and to be able to come back into these communities and help them to set a goal to reach for themselves. . .that makes me feel good."

He discussed his years of addiction. "As the girl was saying, I was one of the fortunate ones. I had parents who loved me. And I always had a purpose in life and knew right from wrong. And even though I was out there abusing, I still had a conscience. I remember getting money to get high, and I would cry all the way there because I knew it wasn't what the Lord put me here for. And I fought it until I put myself together. And I feel damned good about Gregory now, I really do."

None of that got on the air. It wasn't part of the story, although it was a pivotal moment in my own education. At that moment, I knew the real war on AIDS wasn't going to be fought at glamorous star-studded benefit galas hosted by Elizabeth Taylor; it would be fought inside the souls of individuals like Gregory Howard.

In a neighborhood near the downtown Newark Catholic school, children play on the streets during recess. The school can't afford a playground. In plain view of the children, a scantily dressed woman solicited her customer, and climbed into his beat-up Buick. He pushed his hand under her sweater as she matter-of-factly withdrew a syringe and rubber cord from her purse. She injected heroin, gave the customer a blow job, and then settled back, clothing in disarray, and stared apathetically at the ceiling of the car. Her eyes glazed over, her mind soaring in heroin heaven, while the man clumsily fondled and grabbed at her body.

It was noon, on a sunny winter day, and I was standing not ten yards away, watching all this. The prostitute, Shiela, had promised me an interview about AIDS, but told me to wait when she spotted her customer driving down the avenue in front of the Catholic school. I concentrated on what this little episode represented in the context of the epidemic. Shiela was using heroin, had probably shared needles, and was more than likely infected with the AIDS virus. If she had intercourse with her customer, Shiela might pass that virus onto him. And it was likely she serviced several customers a day.

When at last she got out of the car, Shiela wandered down the sidewalk vaguely in my direction. It was obvious she had forgotten all about me. I stopped her, pointed to my tape recorder, and said, "Can I ask you a couple of questions now?" Shiela's face wrinkled up with the effort of trying to figure out who this crazy, white lady with the microphone was. She stared hard at me, and then smiled with recognition and said, "Yeah. You do that." I asked her if she ever shared works.

"No, never, not now."

"Did you in the past?"

"I used to. Quite a while ago. But AIDS became an epidemic and it was like something said, 'Don't share your works.' As far as AIDS is concerned, very few people catch AIDS from needles. They mostly get it from sex. I'm quite sure Liberace wasn't no dope fiend, Rock Hudson wasn't a dope fiend. But still they got it. They didn't share no needles. I'm not saying it doesn't come from needles, but you have less percentage from needles. It's not an excuse. It's just the way I feel."

Most of the junkies I've interviewed have denied being addicts, said they weren't infected with the AIDS virus, swore they no longer shared their works, and brushed off the epidemic as a "homosexual problem." It takes a lot of pushing to get past the denial. So I pushed Shiela, hard. I told her a recent study of heroin users in Newark showed that at least 65 percent were already infected with the AIDS virus. She said that was a shame. I told her over 60 percent of the prostitutes recently tested in Newark were infected. She hadn't heard that one.

"I was not aware of that," she said. "It scares you to death! Any working girl should work with condoms from the beginning. You should never work without a condom, never. Because you're having sex with Tom, Dick and Harry, and who knows what he has. You gotta protect yourself. If you do, you won't have no problem."

The most hopeful group I encountered in Newark were the non-addicted prostitutes, a pragmatic, tough-talking, levelheaded group. They spoke with disdain about their colleagues who use heroin, referring to them often as "ten-dollar Suzies," women desperate for money to buy their next fix, and willing to take $10 for sexual services for which the other women demand a minimum of $50.

On one of Newark's busiest streets at about 3:00 on a Tuesday afternoon, I talked to two hookers in their early thirties. They told me they knew all about AIDS, and carried AIDS leaflets in their pockets. They said they insisted their clients wear condoms. When they talked about condoms the women became very excited, often interrupting each other.

"I tell them to run around to the drug store. . .They say, 'Oh! Well, I don't feel like it.' I say, 'You don't what! And it's right around the corner! You must be crazy!' "

"They don't get the same feeling. C'mon! I tell them, 'You're not gonna get any feeling lyin' on your dyin' bed.' "

In covering AIDS, I have met many prostitutes — gay men in San Francisco, dying women in Tanzania, self-confident hookers in Paris — and I have learned that prostitutes have a very professional attitude about their work. They know how many risks they are willing to take, how much money they expect to earn and what they intend to do with the money. Many, if not most, prostitutes dream of saving their money, eventually accumulating enough cash to buy a home and start a small business. Most American prostitutes I have interviewed have been well informed about AIDS, and, unless they were heroin addicts, were weighing their personal risks carefully.

Africa was another story. Very few African prostitutes make more than 50 cents per client, so most see over a dozen clients a day. They can't afford health care, and most suffer constantly from a variety of sexually transmitted diseases and infections. AIDS has simply added to what was already a public health nightmare.

In Bukoba, Tanzania I met a woman who had worked in Nairobi as a prostitute for two years. She worked hard in the Kenyan capital, and returned to her Lake Victoria town a comparatively wealthy woman.

She bought a home with a plot of land for a vegetable garden, got her children good school clothes, and became a respected Bukoba citizen. That lasted two years. Then she became sick, and came under the care of Bukoba's Dr. Jayo Kidenya. In July 1986, Kidenya took me to the woman's hospital room.

A young woman sat listlessly, barely able to keep upright on her steel frame bed. Kidenya listened patiently as she detailed her medical history. The dark, gray concrete walls enveloped her. A faint odor of human waste filled the small cell. She was beyond caring. She could not have weighed more than 80 pounds; her body had been reduced to mere skeletal dimensions. Her lips were ulcerated and small sores were splotched all over her skin. As she spoke to Dr. Kidenya, her eyes glazed over, and it was obvious she knew she was going to die.

"She says the first sign she noticed was difficulty in getting stools. She felt like going, but nothing came out. She was giving out mucoid material. Two months later it became mixed with blood. And this was associated with severe abdominal pains. She noticed she was getting weaker. The limbs could not carry her body. She could not move her hands. And then she was losing weight. She got fevers. She was having treatment at the dispensary without any relief. She needed help, she went to her mother, and her mother brought her here. And now she has nausea and she vomits."

In a nearby cell, another young woman, Noticia, struggled to sit up for her visitors. She was extremely weak. With the doctor's help, she raised herself and by sheer will stayed erect. She, too, was mere skin and bones. She looked as if she might have once been a beautiful woman, but now her bony face was hard to look at.

"When did Noticia first get sick?"

"In January. In the beginning she noted one abscess on her neck, and later they had spread all over her body. She was weak. And she developed fevers and tightness and coughing. So she came to the hospital."

"How old is she?"

"Twenty-three. She is divorced now for three years and has one child."

"What has she been doing for money?"

She is a typist. After the divorce she was employed by the water company."

"How is the health of her child?"

She says her child is very well."

Outside Noticia's room, I asked Kidenya how she got the disease. He shrugged his shoulders and said it was impossible to know for sure. "But surely it must be heterosexual. She must have gotten it from a man."

When I met these women, I identified with them very strongly. They were the first female AIDS patients I had interviewed, and I felt almost faint in their rooms. When I started covering AIDS in 1981, my heart always went out to the men with AIDS that I interviewed, but I never personally identified with their plight. Meeting Noticia and her fellow hospital patients in Tanzania, however, I found myself imagining I was on that steel-framed death bed, mustering my last bits of strength to sit upright and greet visitors.

Now almost daily I hum to myself the old Phil Ochs tune "There But For Fortune." And I find it increasingly difficult to remain dispassionate and objective in my coverage of the epidemic.

Last year, I had a dinner party for some fellow AIDS reporters during the International AIDS Conference in Washington. Some twenty AIDS reporters gathered in a restaurant dining room, ordered mounds of delicious gourmet food and drank heavily. A journalist friend who does not cover AIDS joined us, and midway through the meal fell uncommonly silent. The next day I asked her why she had been so quiet. "I guess I was blown away by you guys," she said. "I've never been with a group that felt like yours since the time I had dinner with a bunch of former Vietnam war correspondents. You are just like them, with all your gallows humor, heavy drinking, loud partying and closeness. There's a sort of wartime intimacy among you. I guess I was quiet because I found it so fascinating."

Two things keep me going: a sense of duty, and the inspiration I find in small battles fought and won every day. "Information," said Winston Churchill, "is the key to winning a war." As for inspiration, I find it everywhere.

I found courage, humanity and sacrifice in Newark that exceeded anything I had seen in my travels around the world. Take Jean Givens, for example. She is an elderly black woman who has already raised her own family, and works as a security guard at a local school. Givens has taken in seven foster children, four with AIDS.

When I visited Jean Givens, her dining room table was piled high with boxes of Pampers and baby formula. In the living room, a four-year-old girl jumped about the room madly, stopping only to gasp deeply for breath, filling the room with a grating, rasping sound. She obviously adored Jean Givens, and hugged her constantly. In contrast, two tiny infants lay in baby seats, strangely silent and lifeless. They were born with AIDS. As Givens hugged her four-year-old child, she spoke about the seven children she has taken into her home.

"Well, I think other people should do it, really. It's not the children's fault, and it's a shame. We have to face it; AIDS is here. And the children shouldn't have to suffer for it. That's what I really believe. If I had a bigger house I would take more. I really would."

Jean Givens is not alone. Throughout Newark, people have stepped forward with nobility in the city's crisis. Their strength guides them, even when, as in the case of Sylvia, it seems fate has dealt them the worst possible hand. I met Sylvia in her four-year-old daughter's hospital room. The daughter, Rosalia, had AIDS. So did Sylvia. They got the disease from Sylvia's husband, a heroin user, who died last year from the disease. Sylvia's body was so racked by disease that she had to be carried upstairs to Rosalia's room. I asked what made her go on.

"God," she said. "God, he's the only one. Whenever I feel depressed, or angry, I just pray. And ask him, is it fair that this is happening to me? Because I've always been a housewife, I mind my own business, I take care of my kids. And I'm paying the price for something I had nothing to do with. So I always end up praying, asking God to give me strength to keep on. That's what I got to believe in."

Sylvia's last wish was that she would survive to take care of Rosalia. A couple of months after I left Newark, a hospital social worker called to tell me Rosalia was dead. And in October, a late-night caller told me Sylvia had passed away. The news hurt, both times. But I was consoled by the fact that Sylvia's last wish — to outlive her daughter — had come true.

Because I am a trained immunologist, I know what we are up against in this epidemic. I have watched doctors, nurses and researchers burn out, unable to handle the depression and stress involved in dealing with AIDS. Since my trip to Africa, I often ask myself how much longer I can handle the AIDS story. Professionally speaking, AIDS has been very good for me. In purely selfish terms, it has brought me a modicum of fame, the respect of both my colleagues and top scientists and a tremendous amount of intellectual excitement. No story I have covered has been as challenging as AIDS. Or as depressing. But small glimmers of faith have helped me to continue reporting the realities of AIDS.

VII

AIDS Prevention Policies

THIS SECTION PRESENTS perspectives on the development of political strategies to combat AIDS, including critiques of various national AIDS programs, specifically in regard to educational and support services for women. The variety of topics not only demonstrates the complexity of women's AIDS issues, but also the effects of the AIDS epidemic in different regions of the world.

Even though fewer AIDS cases have been reported in Western Europe than the United States, most of these countries have mobilized their social welfare and health systems. These strategies include education in schools (from kindergarten to university), public safe sex campaigns, increased availability of drug treatment programs or easy access to clean needles, and readily available social welfare programs which provide housing, food, and medical care for those who need it.

In Eastern Europe, where few cases have been reported so far, prevention and education is also taken seriously. Besides talking about safe sex in the media, and encouraging the sale and use of condoms, some countries have made additional prevention efforts. In Poland, for example, little stickers with inviting red lips promoting AIDS awareness can be found in many places; and in the fall of 1987, plastic shopping bags carried AIDS prevention messages.

Reading about the impact of AIDS in Latin America, Africa and Asia, one gets the sense that AIDS is just one of many epidemics, an additional burden to the public health care systems. Because treatments for AIDS, even blood screening for HIV, are prohibitively expensive for the budgets of many countries, prevention is taken seriously.

Cash-poor countries do not have the resources to provide health or social services for their people. Many of these countries rely on international organizations for assistance. Several African countries have received help in carrying out their own prevention campaigns. Rather than using the same educational tools as the Europeans, these countries have tried to find the most effective ways of bringing the message of AIDS prevention to their populations.

Song contests, for example, were held in Guinea Bissau, Zaire and Congo. The best songs about AIDS were taped and made available in these countries. For the contest in Guinea Bissau, the U.S. government provided one million condoms to be distributed throughout the country along with the cassettes of the best entries. The winning song ended with the words: "We must be careful; this is the disease of the century; it has such power."

This collection of articles examines the responsibility of the state in regard to public health. It also provides cross cultural glimpses at the role of disease, death and sexuality in different societies.

A Hidden Phenomenon

HELEN JACKSON

Helen Jackson is a lecturer in the School of Social Work at the University of Zimbabwe and is involved in the development of AIDS education and counseling programs.

AIDS IN ZIMBABWE, as in many other African countries, affects women and men more or less equally. And recently the numbers of HIV-positive babies have been on the rise. In Zimbabwe the main modes of transmission are through heterosexual sex and mothers passing the virus on to infants. Blood transfusions are much less significant. In some rural areas the use of unsterile needles might be a factor, but transmission through drug mainlining is probably very rare. Infection by razor blades used by n'angas (traditional healers) is not thought to be a major source of HIV infection, but clients are encouraged to bring their own blades.

The official figure submitted to the World Health Organization (WHO) in October 1987 was 380 cases of AIDS in Zimbabwe, although it was acknowledged at the time that this considerably underrepresented the problem. There is at present no national notification system regarding the numbers of people infected, although different provinces are now trying to establish records. Because AIDS is not considered a "notifiable" disease, data generally comes from limited sources: the Blood Transfusion Service (all blood has been screened for HIV since July 1985); small-scale studies of probable high-risk groups, such as prostitutes and patients at clinics for sexually transmitted diseases; and individual studies and monitoring by concerned doctors and other health workers.

Various studies yield different figures, most of which are not available to the public. Perhaps of most interest and concern are the blood transfusion figures from mid-1985, which indicated that over 2 percent of the 70,000 blood samples tested were found to be HIV-positive; and the figures from a study of a clinic for sexually transmitted diseases in Harare, Zimbabwe's capital, in January 1987 which showed that 18.5 percent of 503 patients screened were HIV-positive. However, there is undoubtedly some risk of false positive results, so figures have to be treated cautiously.

Initially the government's attitude was tentative, and included instructions to doctors not to inform their patients of an AIDS or HIV diagnosis. But during 1987, this began to change significantly. The Ministry of Health launched an AIDS awareness campaign early that year, which targeted not only health workers, but also the population in general. In addition to posters, leaflets and discussion groups, the campaign also included the mass media, with radio and television advertisements and programs, and a series of articles in the major daily newspaper. An AIDS advisory committee called ZAHEC (Zimbabwe AIDS Health Education Committee) has now been established under the Ministry of Health to monitor and spearhead initiatives to control and treat AIDS. One subcommittee focuses specifically on AIDS awareness.

The health care system is making considerable progress in examining the problem of AIDS and seropositivity, particularly with regard to preventive measures. However, health workers, and doctors in particular, still need guidelines for treating people with AIDS, accurate diagnosis of AIDS, counseling of people with AIDS or HIV-related infections, as well as their families and particularly their sexual partners.

Non-governmental agencies and individual social workers could also begin to provide the much needed social and psychological support for people with AIDS. So far, the problem has been viewed as primarily a medical one, and there has been little effective counseling. Indeed, many doctors still tell their patients they have something other than AIDS or HIV-related infections. For example, in the case of someone developing HIV-related tuberculosis, they may be told about tuberculosis, but not its underlying cause.

Nevertheless, many individuals, both inside and outside government, are deeply concerned about AIDS and about the need to develop much more comprehensive services. Church organizations are starting to investigate what role they can play. In 1988, for example, the Catholic Church started a multi-denominational association that is to train counselors. FACT (Family AIDS Counseling Trust) opened in January 1988 to develop training for counselors in the city of Mutare. Research is being initiated at the University of Zimbabwe, at the School of Social Work and within the health sector. Moreover, the government, various organizations, and individuals are trying to promote AIDS awareness around the country — in schools, workplaces, and in a variety of community settings.

Before the Ministry of Health's awareness campaign, a survey investigating AIDS and sexual behavior among young Zimbabweans, conducted by the University of Zimbabwe in January 1987, indicated that even among the better educated, there was great ignorance about AIDS.

These are the attitudes revealed by some women:

"People don't believe it's serious. You can't see it [AIDS]. You won't get men to change their behavior — they all want to go to nightclubs now, and they think even if they get AIDS they can get cured, like other sexually transmitted diseases. They all go to a *n'anga*. *N'angas* say they can cure it, but I don't believe it." — Young seamstress in Harare

"Like with so many other issues, men are going to blame women for AIDS, and I don't think men take the risk seriously." — University lecturer

"I think we're all going to get it anyway, so why worry? We should just enjoy ourselves and forget it. We've probably already got it, so it's too late." — University student

"There are too many other problems here — malnutrition, malaria, diarrhea. How can we focus everything on AIDS? People in the west exaggerate it because it affects them. Look at how much is spent on AIDS research compared with malaria, but how many people die in developing countries from malaria each year compared with AIDS? Or malnutrition? Or get bilharzia? Or don't have clean drinking water?" — Lecturer

"If somebody in the class had AIDS, I wouldn't sit near them. They should have to leave." — Rural high school student

"We want to know more about it, and how we can avoid it. But how do we get information? We need information." — Rural high school student

"If I was HIV-positive, I wouldn't want to know. I wouldn't get tested." — University student

"I don't know it what I've got is AIDS. I don't want to know.

207

I don't want everyone to reject me." — Chronically ill professional

While some of the population is beginning to realize that AIDS is a serious problem, this has not yet led to any serious change of behavior to reduce its spread. Many people do not think the problem relates to them, or that they have any control over it. With growing awareness, there is a considerable risk of a moralistic and repressive backlash against people with AIDS, especially since many people believe that AIDS can be spread by casual social contact.

There are already occasional signs of this, as in a recent advertisement in *The Herald*: "Sex Outside of Marriage is Sin — The Wages of Sin: Death — Heard of AIDS?"

Media coverage of AIDS has been varied and frequent, but articles in the press often relate to other countries, and have the tendency to sensationalize the issues rather than informing. These articles are sometimes too technical, like a series put out by the Ministry of Health, which even some medical students had difficulty in following. Nevertheless, occasionally there has been some good, balanced coverage.

The attitude of the *n'angas* towards AIDS is an area of further confusion. Some have claimed they can cure it, and the head of their umbrella organization, ZINATHA, a university professor, has criticized the Ministry of Health for refuting their claims without first seeking scientific evidence. The relationship between traditional and Western medicine in Zimbabwe is sometimes problematic, but many people respect and utilize both. Cooperation between the *n'angas* and government health workers is crucial in handling AIDS effectively, particularly in view of the many social and emotional problems that arise in addition to the purely medical ones. *N'angas* can undoubtedly play a useful role, provided there is mutual trust, cooperation, and a willingness to learn on both sides.

AIDS in Zimbabwe is still a fairly new phenomenon, and a very hidden one in real, personal terms. Most people don't know anyone with it, or are unaware of it even if they do. Many of those actually suffering from AIDS-related illnesses don't know their diagnosis, and health workers treating them may also be unsure of the underlying cause of infection. Public figures who may have died of AIDS have been reported as having died from other causes. However, in neighboring Zambia, President Kaunda has declared that his son died of AIDS in 1986, and his openness is very encouraging.

Unfortunately, real awareness of the risks of unprotected sex with different partners, and conversely of the non-infectivity of the virus in normal social situations, will lead to behavior change only when many more people are known and seen to be sick with the disease, or are dying because of it. And then there will be the question of whether people in general will extend support, concern and respect for people with AIDS, or whether we will see an intensifying rejection and fear, as shown in a Sunday newspaper headline: "Even worms will shun an AIDS victim's corpse."

A further problem lies in the likely differential attachment of blame and responsibility between women and men. AIDS in Zimbabwe is very much a heterosexual problem, with high-risk individuals including workers separated from a spouse (such as migrant workers and army personnel), prostitutes, prisoners, some refugees, and young single people. The spouses or sexual partners of any of the above will also be at risk, as will future children.

If prejudice about AIDS follows the pattern of beliefs around other sexually transmitted diseases and sexual/reproductive problems, then those likely to receive the most blame and the least support or understanding are female prostitutes, and perhaps women in general. Women are commonly blamed for the birth of a disabled child, for the birth of a daughter when a son was wanted, or for failing to produce children in a marriage — and many women are divorced by men for these reasons. It seems unlikely that women will escape scapegoating over AIDS.

At the same time, women will carry the burden of caring for people with AIDS as an extension of their traditional family roles, but they will be under-represented in the decision-making structures and in the higher echelons of the medical service and other relevant institutions.

Nevertheless, women will have to take the lead in promoting safe sex practices, by refusing casual sexual relationships at all, especially without condoms. They might have to limit actual sexual activities to safer practices. Condoms are widely scorned, at least in public, and it will take a dramatic shift in men's attitudes to use them consistently. Women might be more easily motivated to use them, because they have more to lose (unwanted pregnancy as well as infection). Condoms, of course, do not provide full protection, particularly with the risk of first world countries dumping inferior brands on the third world. Alternative sexual activity or fewer relationships are likely to be safer strategies than condom use alone.

It is too soon to say how attitudes towards AIDS in Zimbabwe will develop over time, but it is unfortunately only too clear that it will be very difficult to achieve the necessary changes in sexual behavior to avert an epidemic of crisis proportions. It is also difficult to predict what strategies the government will adopt to monitor, prevent and treat HIV infections and AIDS. Hopefully it will take a lead in promoting the support and integration of people with AIDS, rather than fostering people's prejudices and fears by advocating quarantine, isolation, or forcible testing. Undoubtedly, the next few years will be crucial.

The attitude of foreign governments, agencies and international organizations will also be critical. Zimbabwe, like other developing countries, needs many kinds of support, and it does not help that Africa in general is being scapegoated as the epicenter of the pandemic. The researchers themselves are still debating the origins of AIDS. A more objective, and also more sensitive, approach is needed to assist countries such as Zimbabwe, one which respects and supports local and national initiatives, ideas and developmental strategies.

AIDS Brigade:
Organizing Prevention

NAOMI SCHAPIRO

*Naomi Schapiro is a nurse working in San Francisco. She is a
member of the Nicaraguan AIDS Education Project, which
provides financial and technical assistance for AIDS
education in Nicaragua.*

LAST WEEK AT the city clinic
where I work, a sixty-year-old Salvadoran woman came in desperately
looking for her doctor. She had submitted all of her documentation,
hoping to qualify for permanent residence under the new amnesty
law, only to find out that she also had to provide her HIV antibody
status. I translated into Spanish the complicated consent form for a
confidential, but not anonymous, test, going over her legal protec-
tions and discussing her risk factors. She responded that she had
received a transfusion thirty-five years ago, with the birth of her last
child. Sex? Her husband has been dead for six years. After patiently
listening to my explanations, she stared at me when I asked her to
print and sign her name. "But I never learned how to write, only to
sign my name."

As I spelled her name out so she could laboriously print it over her
beautiful signature, it struck me again that AIDS only puts the
sickness of our society into sharper focus. Our government is spending millions of dollars, which could be spent on AIDS, to create
refugees in Central America. Then it thinks it's preventing the spread
of AIDS by spending more money to test an elderly, illiterate refugee
with no risk factors for the disease.

And here I am, collaborating by carrying out so-called confidential
tests — to which I am very much opposed — because this woman will
get deported if I don't help her to comply. It is precisely this kind of
contradiction that makes me want to go back to Nicaragua. There, in
the midst of an economic and diplomatic struggle for its survival, and
without a single reported case of AIDS, an AIDS education program
has begun that puts our government's prevention efforts to shame.

In November 1987, I stood in a thickly carpeted, air-conditioned room, decorated in modern Scandinavian style, watching my friend, Marsha, demonstrate the stretching ability of a condom. The room was packed with attentive health care providers, using either headsets for translation or clustering around interpreters. She could have been presenting a talk about AIDS prevention at any conference center in the world. But outside, the hot sun, the lake, the volcanos, the empty shells of buildings, ruined in an earthquake and never repaired, reminded us that we could only be in Managua, Nicaragua's capital.

The next day, the independent newspaper *Nuevo Diario* opened its reporting on the conference with this sentence: "Although it might be uncomfortable to accept, if you are one of the people who engage in anal, vaginal or oral sex without a condom, you are a member of one of the groups at higher risk for contracting AIDS." No preaching, no euphemisms, and no disclaimers that AIDS won't spread into the "general population." The article was complete, objective and typical of the Nicaraguan approach to a problem.

In 1979, the Sandinista Liberation Front succeeded in overthrowing Anastasio Somoza Debayle, the last member of a dynasty that controlled Nicaragua with an iron and greedy fist for almost fifty years. Somoza sold vaccines that were donated to his country's children and pocketed relief money that poured into Nicaragua after the 1972 earthquake destroyed most of downtown Managua. Because of the Somoza regime's legacy of poverty and disarray, the Sandinistas made improvements in social services their first priority. In order to reduce childhood diseases, they trained community volunteers to be health *brigadistas*. These volunteers took the census of all children under the age of five in their neighborhoods, picked a particular day, and then mobilized the rest of the community to make sure all the children got vaccinated. Using these methods, they eradicated polio within two years and greatly reduced the incidence of measles.

Nicaraguans refer to their revolution as a little girl, now age eight, and brought up to think she can do anything she puts her mind to. The U.S. economic blockade, while creating hardships and shortages, also spurs people on to greater creativity in their solutions to the many problems.

A steady stream of international visitors has poured into Nicaragua to witness this transformation. Many of us go to Nicaragua because there our work is valued. As a nurse in the United States, I alternate between feeling like a band-aid and a safety valve in a system that is ready to explode from its own inadequacies. In Nicaragua, our knowledge of prevention is welcomed and accepted. Then it is evaluated for its relevance by people determined to make their own decisions.

Among the visitors, some of us are gay. In 1984, I made my first trip together with six other lesbians, hoping that we would meet openly gay Nicaraguans. It took some courage to ask a new Nicaraguan friend, who was sweet and never came on to us, if he was gay. He assured us that he was not. On my second trip, in 1986, my friend told me that he had in fact started going to gay bars and had had relationships with men. This process of gradual opening up has been mirrored all over Nicaragua.

In 1986, I participated in a tour of Bay Area health workers. We were co-sponsored by the Victoria Mercado Brigade — named for a murdered Chicana, lesbian union activist — and the Harvey Milk Democratic Club. The previous year, the first Victoria Mercado Construction Brigade had sent a group of gays and lesbians to Managua to build a community center. This time, we went to present information about AIDS at a health conference and to members of the gay community. This project was dedicated to the memory of Bill Kraus, a gay rights activist also involved in solidarity work with Central America, who died of AIDS.

We gave presentations at an annual U.S.-Nicaragua Health Colloquium, at medical schools and at teaching hospitals in a couple of cities. One of the project members gave safe sex workshops for gay and bisexual men. These presentations sparked the interest of Dr. Leonel Argüello, the epidemiology director for the Ministry of Health (MINSA). When we returned to San Francisco, we founded the Nicaragua AIDS Education Project, in order to send technical and financial assistance to MINSA and to our contacts in the gay community.

Meanwhile, some of the Nicaraguans we had met during the tour began conducting their own safe sex workshops within the gay community and giving general prevention talks in some of Managua's secondary schools. This is not always an easy task. Nicaragua is a predominantly Catholic country, with its own brand of homophobia. There have never been laws against homosexuality in Nicaragua, either under Somoza or under the Sandinistas. But discrimination is widespread, even though violence against gays is rare. There are, as yet, no public gay organizations.

Most Nicaraguans live with their extended families, sleeping in the same room as their relatives, having little privacy. There are bars with a gay flavor, but as the war wears on, people can't afford to go out much. Nevertheless, gay activists have started to meet, motivated, to some extent, by the threat of an AIDS epidemic. They have two major fears: first, that they will contract AIDS if they don't learn to protect themselves, and second, that AIDS will somehow fuel an anti-gay backlash.

MINSA, which had a functioning AIDS Commission before the United States did, began to work on the issue. AIDS was not a top priority in Nicaragua then; there are many more pressing health needs. But the threat exists, and under the current circumstances, an AIDS epidemic would stretch the scarce resources beyond their limitations. There is only one solution: prevention through education. This is a realistic goal, since health educators have gained valuable experiences in previous popular health campaigns.

The AIDS Commission published a full-page ad in the Sandinista newspaper, with explicit information about both transmission and prevention of AIDS. It also printed an informational flyer to pass out to the general population. Five thousand ELISA test kits were donated, and every hemophiliac in the country was tested, as well as a number of volunteers.

As of July 13, 1988, five Nicaraguans have turned up seropositive. MINSA has located twenty-one seropositive foreigners. Rather than expelling or quarantining them, they were advised to "take care" of themselves and the Nicaraguans around them. Blood is checked for the HIV antibody in the central blood bank in Managua. However, most blood transfusions take place in field hospitals in the war zones, where screening is not available.

The chief architect of this nascent program, Leonel Argüello, had visited San Francisco in July 1987, where he was surprised and impressed by the massive participation of openly lesbians and gay men in every AIDS program in the city. As a result of his visit, Argüello, who has been promoted to vice minister of health, began speaking publicly about high-risk practices, rather than high-risk groups. Because of his openness towards a grassroots campaign, he accepted the gay volunteers' proposal to work with them directly in the planning and development of this AIDS education and prevention program. He also stressed the fact that all Nicaraguans, regardless of their sexual orientation and practices, have a right to honest information and health care. This proposal was approved by the Minister of Health, Commandante Dora Maria Tellez, who opened a press conference in Nicaragua by handing out condoms to journalists.

I returned to Nicaragua for a third time in November 1987, as part of a group of Bay Area health workers involved in AIDS service organizations. The contra war had bled the country for six years and the economy was a disaster. Inflation was rampant. Our suitcases were laden with gifts of cooking oil, toothpaste, sanitary napkins, and lubricated condoms. Basic food supplies and gasoline were rationed, and the generous loan of a friend's car meant getting up at 6:00 a.m. to wait in line for gas and scouring the city for motor oil. Friends who had paid for my dinner the year before could scarcely afford to pay for their own drinks. And the letters I mailed from Managua had their front as well as their back completely covered with stamps.

But devastating as the economic changes were, exciting developments had occurred. As a result of the gay volunteers' proposal, there was now a functioning team of gay advisors working directly with MINSA on the AIDS education and prevention program. Together they were working to found the first national Center for Sexual Education and Information. Specifics of the plan included a telephone hotline, a resource library and a training course for health educators and volunteers. The focus was to be not only on AIDS, but also on other sexually transmitted diseases, and all aspects of sexuality.

The major focus of the trip was our renewed participation in the annual U.S.-Nicaragua Health Colloquium. This time, an entire morning of the conference was devoted to AIDS. Scattered throughout the audience was the first batch of volunteer health workers, who had just started training. We later went to their first formal training session, which involved small group discussions and role playing. Suddenly we realized that the building we were in was being fumigated. We poured outside into the courtyard, coughing and choking. We finished the workshop and ate pizza while a nurse from MINSA, who up until then had never met an openly gay person, passed out Japanese "Love Time" condoms to a teenage *afeminado* (queen), and looked curiously at pictures in a gay magazine.

Now I am back home, and sometimes that courtyard, the lakes and the volcanos seem like part of a dream. But letters keep arriving to tell us of the continuing progress of the program and to request more condoms — lubricated only, please. The collective of health educators — an equal number of women and men — have continued their training and have begun to give workshops under the auspices of MINSA. At the urging of the gay health *brigadistas*, MINSA solicited the cooperation of the police to allow an AIDS prevention workshop in the Central Park, one of Managua's cruising areas. About twenty men attended that workshop. We, here in the United States, are responding to the proposal of MINSA and the collective, trying to raise $10,000 to fund the Center for Sexual Education and Information for its first six months. So far Nicaragua is the only Central American country that is trying to prevent the spread of the AIDS epidemic. In one tiny country the course of this devastating disease may be changed, because a government and a people know how to work together.

Reaching Within, Reaching Out

MARIE MARTHE SAINT CYR-DELPE

*In 1983, the CDC classified Haitians as an AIDS risk group —
together with gay men, IV drug users and hemophiliacs. This
classification was withdrawn in April 1985, but by that time
serious damage had already been done to the Haitian
communities domestically and abroad. In the United
States, social ostracism and increased discrimination
against Haitians has occurred.*

*Marie Marthe Saint Cyr-Delpe currently with WARN, worked
for the Haitian Coalition on AIDS, a New York City-funded
social service agency, which provides advocacy and education for
the Haitian community affected by AIDS. About 300 Haitians,
mostly men, have been diagnosed with AIDS in New York. In
Haiti, according to WHO, there have been 1,374 reported AIDS
cases, as of March 1988. In 1983, 12 percent of these cases were
among women, but by 1987 the percentage of cases of women
with AIDS had increased to 40 percent.*

*Marie Marthe Saint Cyr-Delpe has worked as a social worker
within the Haitian community in Pennsylvania, Florida and
New York for many years. She visits friends and relatives in
Haiti regularly. Shortly after her last visit, in January 1988, she
wrote this account.*

Have you ever felt pain stirring deep within
when you are unable to pinpoint the whys and wherefore of
its existence?
Have you ever wanted to undo what is done
to you
to those you have learned to love
regardless of the cause or the reason?

If only I could,
I would have given Janice her mother back,
her father too.

She lays like a limp corpse, folded in my arms
the tears and the wails endlessly flowing
She cried and so did I.

FOR ONCE, I could no longer be everyone's support. While sitting at the kitchen sink, I began to wonder what would become of Janice, this nine-year-old, whom I mothered for twelve months.

Janice was now alone. Three years earlier, her mother was buried in Haiti. She died of a mysterious illness, which had been diagnosed as a different ailment with each recurrence. Janice learned to adapt to her wandering father, a truly adventurous and revolutionary man — in his nationalist ideals as well as in his child-raising attempts. Now her father also lies in his morbid bed of covered pebbles and stones — silent.

I have not seen Janice since.

When I went back home, I stayed busy all the time. I realized that I was afraid, but I didn't dare voice my fear. In the midst of accusations of being disease carriers, uncertain of our own risks, I was afraid to speak the unfamiliar. To speak the unfamiliar in our country is to beckon its curse upon you.

We knew so little about AIDS. Accused by those who profess to know all, one begins to doubt one's own knowledge and awareness. I left my job and my town and came to New York. I had been offered work with the Haitian Coalition on AIDS.

As a woman, I had learned early in life that I must be silent, and that demanding was for men; as women, we learn to negotiate our demands through subtle means. AIDS demanded open, pointed negotiations leading to change, a skill I didn't have. I felt that I could no longer live my sexuality. Yet, harboring the same feelings of false security as many others, I saw myself as one with few worries. After all, I am a one-man woman. Unfortunately, for long enough, my partner believed in having as many women as he could get his hands on. I seriously began to worry about my own survival. I remember threatening to kill him if he ever gave me this virus. Our conversations on the subject gave me no real guarantees, but they did give me some sense of assurance that he was concerned. I would fool myself into believing he would be faithful. Of course I hope that he is.

The AIDS crisis has brought forth a twisted interpretation of the role of Haitian women in the transmission of the virus. During my last visit to Haiti in December 1987 to January 1988, I was eager to talk to Haitian people from all walks of life about their perception of the unspoken disease. In the cities of Petion Ville and Port-Au-Prince, the overwhelming attitude among those I spoke to was that women were responsible for the transmission of this disease — blaming the victim among the victims. This attitude prevails in the male/female.interaction in Haiti and among Haitians in diaspora.

Haitian society has so many deficiencies. Success in that society is defined by one's ability to speak the elite language. There are very few employment opportunities or other means to prove oneself. Male sexuality has become a substitute for the social and economic rewards that are lacking. The political and economic hardships have diluted traditional values and allowed violations of social codes. If one sees AIDS transmission as a reflection of the market economy, devised to sustain male economic and sexual power as well as social control, it is not surprising that women are used as scapegoats.

The women with whom I have worked are infected because their husbands are or were bisexuals. In the spirit of self-sacrifice, a highly valued attribute in Haitian family life, these women have maintained their silence. Their anger often is veiled behind a shield of undue commitment, and they are embedded in their prescribed roles. They maintain a passive and subdued facade. Very few have opted to leave these threatening relationships behind them.

I am reminded of Alice. Ever since her husband was told that he was HIV-positive, he had taken to sleeping on the floor. This was before she understood the possibility that she may already be infected or learned the basics of safer sex. She looks fine, and sometimes she forgets all about AIDS. She gets very angry out of sheer frustration at the absence of sexual expression in her life. Generally, she does not talk about her sexuality; she is not used to thinking in terms of her own satisfaction, so she silently accepts her husband's decision to abstain. She finds herself lost in the depth of her own silent fears and hopelessness. And because her self-image is determined by her ability to have and raise children, she was confronted by the worst nightmare of life when her baby died of AIDS.

The greatest pain I have experienced is the lack of concern from the Haitian leadership about the reality of AIDS among us. This lack of concern has some correlation to mores, traditions and trends. Traditionally, the contributions of Haitian women to the country, and to the economic and social survival of the family unit, plagued by male absenteeism, have not been acknowledged. The AIDS crisis can do only one thing among Haitian women: awaken them from their state of self-neglect and self-sacrifice, and develop strong advocates for the promotion of the well-being of the whole family.

Asserting myself is still a struggle, but I remind myself that I must always communicate my needs, and actively define and shape my life. I am no longer silent.

An Active Approach

NICOLINE TAMSMA

*Nicoline Tamsma is a psychologist, a member of the Dutch
Women's AIDS Network, and is currently working at the Office
of Lesbian and Gay Concerns of the Rotterdam Municipal
Health Service. As of December 1987 there were 420 reported
AIDS cases in the Netherlands, 11 of which were women
and 4 were girls; by May 1988, the total number of
cases had increased to 501.*

General AIDS Policy in the Netherlands

WHEN FORMULATING its AIDS
policy in 1983, the Dutch Ministry of Health, Education and Welfare
attached great importance to establishing close links with those
organizations connected to the groups considered to be at risk at that
time. Therefore, in 1984, a team of policy-makers was formed, bringing together experts on IV drug use, health care officials, and
representatives of gay organizations. The team advised the Dutch
government on AIDS issues and was thought to be on the forefront of
AIDS policy. It also coordinated all activities regarding education,
prevention and care.

Until 1987, AIDS education was focused mainly on the separate
risk groups. They received detailed information on how to prevent
HIV infection, and special programs were designed to stimulate behavior change. Most activities were organized by and for homosexual
and bisexual men. COC, Netherlands' largest gay and lesbian organization, worked together with the Amsterdam gay health service and
the national gay and lesbian counseling service.

Their activities were approved and partly funded by the government. Thus gay men could be educated in a non-moralistic way and
according to their specific needs. Since each of the three gay organizations had its own representative in the national policy team, gay
liberation issues were always a matter of concern to the team, which
was chaired by a gay physician.

Meanwhile, the education of the general public took a totally different course. The policy team was very worried about the possible

scapegoating of homosexuals and the rise of widespread panic. However, their interpretation of Dutch epidemiological data also led them to presume that the spread of the virus into the population would occur at a much slower rate than in the United States.

As a result, the general public was given only very basic information of a reassuring nature. People who wanted to know more could turn to various public health organizations for additional advice. This meant that they had to take active steps to obtain detailed facts. On the other hand, members of the risk groups received extensive education without having to take any initiative. This education procedure was called the "active-passive policy."

In spring 1987, this policy was changed. The estimated numbers of HIV-infected among the non-drug-using heterosexual population — even though still very small — started to rise. An extensive education project started, followed by a nationwide campaign to encourage the use of condoms.

Both campaigns tried to avoid moralistic issues, although HIV transmission through sexual contact was too frequently put into the context of promiscuity. But in comparison to campaigns in neighboring countries, such as West Germany or Britain, the Dutch people got more down-to-earth and less fear-inducing information.

The further spread of the HIV virus brought an increased concern among mainstream health organizations and the government. The Secretary of State for Health Affairs wanted more direct influence on AIDS policy and ordered the policy team to be replaced with a national advisory board. Although some members of the policy team were nominated for this board, most nominees held important positions in state affairs, health care or at universities.

The board was to be made up of experts on all the issues relevant to AIDS — ranging from clinical care to homosexuality and from nursing to prostitution. Although the board now has fifteen members, including five women, an expert on special women's issues is lacking.

The Beginning of the Women's AIDS Network

In the summer of 1985, the Dutch prostitutes' organization, Red Thread, joined hands with several women working on AIDS issues to organize the first workshop on women and AIDS at a lesbian health conference in Amsterdam. The workshop participants discussed the need to increase knowledge of women's AIDS issues as soon as possible.

The education strategy of the Dutch policy team withheld information from women: they considered women not to be at a special risk, so that the passive policy used for the general public was applied to women. But since the virus could be transmitted through heterosexual contact, female partners of bisexual men, hemophiliacs or male IV drug users were at risk and had to be educated before it was too late. Another alarming tendency was the growing stigmatization of prostitutes, caused by irrational fears surrounding heterosexual transmission of the virus.

Plans for a national women's AIDS network were drawn up. Women working in various AIDS-related disciplines had to be brought together, not only to provide support, but also to gather as much expertise as possible to criticize and influence official policies and research programs and to work toward better education for women.

Within a few months, women working with Red Thread, the national AIDS hotline, a gay and lesbian counseling service, two women's health centers, and the Municipal Health Authorities of the cities of Amsterdam and Rotterdam formed the network. They were later joined by many others working at the National Association of People with AIDS, addiction centers, AIDS clinics, and so on.

Activities and Ideas

One of the network's essential concerns is the gathering and spreading of up-to-date information, and the first concrete step towards this was the writing and distribution of a brochure on women and AIDS. Arranging the recent facts in an understandable way was relatively easy compared to the struggle for funding and permission to print the brochure.

The AIDS policy team opposed the publishing of a brochure on women and AIDS, arguing that by doing so, women might come to think of themselves as being at risk simply because of their sex. The policy team stated that women could get all the necessary information from the basic brochure for the general public.

A long, sometimes emotional, discussion arose between policymakers and the women's network. The network stressed several points: First, most women would probably not even read a general brochure because of AIDS' image as a gay male disease. Second, the general brochure did not contain enough specific information to answer women's questions about sexual transmission, artificial insemination, mother-to-child transmission, and so forth. Third, and maybe the most important, the persistent emphasis on risk groups was misleading. People are at risk for HIV infection because of their behavior, not because of their group identity. In addition, social groups can never be strictly marked off, certainly not when it comes to sex, which crosses all boundaries.

It took half a year of discussion before the brochure could be presented to the public in the summer of 1986. Never before had the text of an AIDS brochure been so critically looked at, nor had health officials ever attached so many conditions to its distribution. Among women and others working on AIDS issues, the brochure was very well received.

The network's warning about the dangers of heterosexual transmission became evident after the WHO's AIDS Conference in Washington, D.C. in June 1987. Epidemiological data from several parts of the world alarmed not only the Dutch authorities, but also the Dutch press. The Netherlands had discovered that AIDS was a non-gay disease. Authorities and the media started to focus on prostitutes as the source of transmission of the virus to the heterosexual world. For the sake of convenience, they ignored the difference between female IV drug users, who prostitute themselves in order to be able to pay for their addiction, and non-using prostitutes.

In order to respond to this scapegoating, the network organized a press conference, attacking the official passive-active education policy and stressing the need to focus on risk behavior rather than risk groups. They asked the government to put up a realistic, non-moralistic education campaign and to encourage condom use, and they criticized the lack of adequate services for seropositive women or women with AIDS.

The press picked up some of these messages, and as a by-product of the press conference, the network and its brochure became better known. From all over the country, requests for lectures on women and AIDS issues started coming in, and the policy-makers eventually took the network and its opinions more seriously.

As a next step, several women from the network contributed articles to national newspapers and magazines. In 1987, the leading feminist monthly, *Opzij*, published four articles written by women from the network. That way, the network was able to express its ideas to the general public, which was another way to put pressure on the policy-makers. The articles were also meant to start discussions among women about condom use, the possibilities of enjoying safe sex, and the positive and negatives sides of HIV antibody testing.

The network's major concern was still the policy-makers' neglect of women's issues and their focus on women merely as "objects" that could potentially pass on the virus to men and children. In discussions of mother-to-child transmission, the psychological and social needs of HIV-positive women were grossly overlooked.

The network tried to point out that recommending abortions to seropositive women could have serious effects. A woman would have to cope not only with the knowledge that she was infected with the virus, but also with the abortion itself, and the fact that because of her seropositivity she would have to give up the idea of ever becoming a mother.

IV drug use is already the main cause for HIV infection among women in the Netherlands, so official attitudes towards IV drug-using women are critically observed. Some measures taken by the Dutch government to combat the spread of the HIV virus among IV drug users are quite effective: needle exchange and methadone programs are in operation in most larger cities, and they are responsible for the fact that transmission in the Netherlands has slowed down, compared to other European countries.

But IV drug-using women who also work as prostitutes have been labeled "the sting of the AIDS epidemic." It is very striking to note the lack of concern expressed by health officials for the needs of these women, compared to the high interest in the well-being of their male customers.

While fear of increasing homophobic tendencies in the general public has been a main issue in both policy-making and in the designing of various education campaigns, negative reactions towards prostitutes, both drug-using and non-using, seem to be of little concern. The women's AIDS network has repeatedly warned against the scapegoating of prostitutes, as well as against the accompanying pleas for monogamy.

After repeated requests from the network, the Dutch national service organization for family planning and sex education promised to help women who want support in matters concerning their relationships and/or sexuality. Seropositive women who either were or still are IV drug users have access to two organizations providing services for drug addicts in Amsterdam.

On the whole, however, many problems surrounding services for women stem from the fact that AIDS organizations were set up by gay men and have specialized in meeting their needs. Although women are working in some of these organizations, most care providers are men, and most expertise is focused on gay men's needs. Even if these organizations chose to start providing services for women, they would have to hire more women and provide additional training on women's issues.

Plans for the Future

During the first two years of its existence, the network has accomplished a lot, but much more remains to be done. The first women and AIDS brochure, published in 1986, was revised in 1987, and undoubtedly, a third version will follow.

Since the active-passive education policy was abandoned by health officials, it is easier to get permission and funding to publish informational material targeting specific groups. Brochures on the topics of lesbians and AIDS, and pregnancy and AIDS have been prepared. Furthermore, the government subsidized the Dutch translation of Diane Richardson's *Women and the AIDS Crisis* (Pandora Press, London, 1987). In cooperation with a local health care organization, funding for a safe sex workshop for women was secured.

The women from the network will continue to contribute to the media. The network has encouraged health educators to recognize their responsibility to give general matter-of-fact information on women and AIDS. Lectures on more specific or political issues will continue to be a project of the network.

Unfortunately, the network's time and energy are somewhat limited. Although over twenty women have joined the organization, their work on women and AIDS issues are additions to their already heavy work schedules. Many group members are also engaged professionally in other demanding AIDS work. The coordination, administration and finances of the network become more complex with expansion.

The network has asked the Dutch government to subsidize a small staff consisting of one coordinator and one secretary. If the government agrees, the staff will be working out of a women's health center in Utrecht, the fourth largest city in the Netherlands. This will unite the network with the women's health movement, and it will encourage collaboration on AIDS issues within the movement.

Turning Issues Upside Down

KATHERINE FRANKE

Katherine Franke is an attorney working for the AIDS Anti-Discrimination Unit of New York City's Human Rights Commission.

The LESBIAN/GAY and women's rights movements have stood for many things. Perhaps most importantly, they have allowed both women and men to think expansively about the ways in which we express ourselves sexually. They are also responsible for raising public consciousness on contraceptive methods and reproductive technology, as well as challenging us all to think of new ways to manifest our sexuality beyond traditional female/male models.

In many regards, AIDS has stopped these movements in their tracks. For that matter, the epidemic of stigma surrounding AIDS has given many people license to seek refuge in racist, classist, sexist, homophobic and xenophobic notions of moral superiority. As a result, in fighting these two facets of the AIDS epidemic — both the virus and its accompanying stigma — many of us find ourselves addressing prejudice for which a new-found "scientific" legitimacy has emerged. The difficult thing about fighting the good fight in the AIDS arena, however, is that very often AIDS turns traditional arguments of justice and fairness on their heads. This is particularly the case when discussing the effect of HIV on reproductive rights and women's choices of sexual expression.

Women with AIDS or HIV infection have been judged as bad mothers and wives, or simply as bad women, because they are viewed in the media and in the minds of many Americans as the vectors by which HIV is transmitted to men or children. Rather than looking at HIV infection as a threat to a woman's own future health, it is explained in terms of the other people in her life who she is thought to have put in danger.

Prenatal HIV antibody testing is never conducted in a social or political vacuum. These testing policies interact with civil and criminal laws in ways that further render women "guilty of HIV infection." Obviously, widespread testing of any kind makes sense only when it has some positive effect upon public health, particularly the health of those being tested. HIV antibody testing, on the contrary, has quite often led to coerced abortions, loss of child custody, and a whole host of related discrimination, but it rarely slows the spread of HIV. Few resources have been allocated to the education of women about transmission prevention. Given the social context surrounding HIV antibody testing, it can only be viewed as punishment, not as prevention.

Examining the effects of HIV-related infections upon reproductive rights, it becomes clear how this retrovirus has brought out retro-values in many people. Traditionally, the state has articulated an interest in preserving and protecting so-called fetal rights. This allegedly compelling interest was demonstrated most clearly in the 1973 *Roe v. Wade* decision in which the U.S. Supreme Court recognized a woman's right to choose an abortion. In reaching its decision, the court found it appropriate to weigh a woman's right to privacy against the state's interest in protecting the future life of the fetus. In short, the court determined that a state may bar an "elective abortion" by asserting a compelling interest in the potential life of the fetus at viability.

Those who seek to defend "fetal rights" have looked to *Roe v. Wade* in support of efforts to forcibly subject a pregnant woman to a Caesarean section over her objections; to place governmental restraints on a pregnant woman's physical activities, diet and lifestyle; and to hold mothers liable for injuries to children caused by "prenatal negligence."

This compelling state interest in fetal survival seems to evaporate when the mother and/or fetus have been exposed to HIV. When HIV infections become a factor in the abortion decision, the state's duty to defend potential life shifts to the interest of protecting society from the possibility of another person with AIDS. Here, as elsewhere, AIDS turns the issue on its head.

This abandonment of the fight to protect the lives of HIV-positive babies cannot be divorced from the moral judgments passed upon anyone who tests positive. In the minds of many Americans, these women are bad women, and will be bad mothers, because they are perceived to be either prostitutes or IV drug users. As such, they are responsible for their HIV infection. Conversely, heterosexual, white, middle-class women are more frequently viewed as the "innocent victims" of secretly bisexual men in their lives. It is to these women that most government-sponsored prevention education has been directed.

When determining the extent to which the state should intervene to protect "future life," we seem to feel differently about this moral duty when we consider parents who have engaged in so-called bad behavior. In some cities, it is routine practice in the public hospitals to run toxicology tests on poor pregnant women who are admitted for delivery. If the tests reveal the presence of any "street drugs," this fact will be reported to the child protective services authorities, at which time the responsibility shifts to the mother to show that she is a fit mother in light of her demonstrated illicit drug use. Obviously, HIV antibody testing raises the stakes for mothers who test positive — those with control over her continued custody of her children. AFDC or the like, make the assumption that she is either an IV drug user or a prostitute, and either way she will probably die soon anyway.

Accordingly, our interest in protecting the lives of fetuses potentially infected with HIV is diminished to the extent that we judge or stigmatize their parents for the bad behavior we assume they engaged in. This stigma is far more infectious than HIV, since virtually all children born to HIV-positive women suffer stigma regardless of their own antibody status. In many settings, babies born to HIV-positive parents are presumed to be carrying the virus and are next to impossible to place in foster care. Indeed, these so-called "innocent victims" or "most tragic victims" of AIDS receive society's opprobrium despite their "innocence." As a result, often we find politicians who have otherwise opposed abortion encouraging HIV-infected women to abort their babies. Again, AIDS turns the debate on its head.

Many states and the federal government encourage, and in some instances require, pregnant women to undergo HIV antibody testing. As is the case with most HIV antibody testing programs, those recommending testing have not adequately explained the importance of the test as a public health tool in a given context. More often than not, proponents of prenatal HIV testing recommend the test so that "she can know her options." Rarely, if ever, do these people acknowledge that the only option they are talking about is abortion. Ironically, many of those who favor prenatal HIV testing have been vocal opponents of abortion, and as such have had a difficult time saying the "A" word in this context. As discussed below, seemingly simple solutions like antibody testing do not answer the complex questions presented by both AIDS epidemics, one created by stigma, and the other created by a virus.

The simultaneous debates over the right of a woman to choose an abortion and the right of the state to encourage HIV-infected women to abort are being played out in very cruel terms on the state level across the country. In all fifty states, confirmed cases of AIDS must be reported to state public health officials. In several states seropositivity must also be reported to state health officials. In addition, several states have already enacted laws criminalizing willful transmission of HIV. Fourteen other states have similar bills pending in their legislatures, some of which would make it a crime for a person who tests HIV-positive to have sexual intercourse. Various law enforcement officials have tried to use these laws in cases of biting, spitting, and blood donation as well as sexual transmission. If a person could be regarded as a criminal under these circumstances, surely it would be a crime for a woman who tests HIV-positive to carry her child to term. It is conceivable that in those states that deem HIV infection a reportable disease, the state could require hospitals, doctors and family planning clinics to run a check on any pregnant woman they treat.

Similarly, where state legislatures or courts are willing to impose civil liability for willful or negligent transmission of HIV, it is conceivable that an HIV-positive child may sue her mother and/or father for exposing her to HIV. Furthermore, it is imaginable that pregnant HIV-positive women, as well as pregnant women with AIDS, will be forced to take AIDS or HIV-related medication for the benefit of the fetus. More often than not, these treatments have questionable efficacy in treating AIDS-related infections, while having demonstrated adverse side effects. As new drugs are developed, it is possible that children born to HIV-positive women will be able to sue their mothers for refusal to undergo these treatments prenatally.

In many states, a poor woman can receive Medicaid funding only for "therapeutic" abortions, that is, only when she can show that continuing to term will endanger her own life or the life of her baby, or when she can demonstrate that the baby will be "deformed." Pro-choice groups have fought these narrow restrictions on publicly funded abortions, arguing that the state should pay for all poor women's abortions independent of the reasons why they seek to terminate their pregnancies. State restrictions on abortion funding amounts to limiting a poor woman's ability to exercise her rights recognized in *Roe v. Wade*.

HIV infection further complicates this policy debate. Various state public health officials have stated that a fetus infected with HIV would be considered deformed for the purposes of state Medicaid abortion regulations. For the time being, however, there is no test that can show prenatally that a baby of an HIV-infected mother has been infected as well. Indeed, assuming for the moment that a pregnant woman who tests HIV-positive is truly carrying HIV, and that there is a meaningful nexus between HIV and AIDS, there is only a 30 to 50 percent chance that she will pass the virus to her child. Even where prenatal transmission does occur, there is no guarantee that the HIV-positive baby will ever get sick. When compared with the other fetal tests which qualify a woman for abortion funding on account of fetal disability, maternal HIV testing is an extremely unreliable predictor of future infant health.

Similarly, many public health officials have also cited as credible recent medical rumors suggesting that pregnancy can trigger the onset of opportunistic infections for some women who have been exposed to HIV. In other words, carrying a baby to term may endanger the life of a mother who has been exposed to HIV, and may, as a result, entitle her to a state-funded abortion. While it is, in many regards, a good thing that HIV-positive women will qualify for Medicaid-funded abortions, it is important to recognize that this result will not be achieved because of the state's respect for woman's right to make reproductive choices. Rather, this right will be secured as a result of the state's diminished interest in the life of the potentially HIV-infected fetus, often offensively called the "AIDS baby."

The significance of maternal HIV infection, and the concomitant assumption of fetal infection, vis-à-vis state-funded abortion, must be seen in the light of the public sentiment favoring abortions of HIV-infected fetuses, as manifested in directive counseling which HIV-infected mothers often receive. Most likely, state legislatures will not begin moving toward compelled abortions for HIV-positive mothers. However, given the coercive nature of prenatal counseling received by HIV-positive women, the distinction between abortions mandated by law and abortions coerced by physician counseling will, in reality, become a distinction without a difference.

Coercive pregnancy counseling for HIV-positive women must be contrasted with other prenatal genetic tests, which are usually very expensive but truly voluntarily administered. As such, they are primarily used by middle-class women who can pay for them. In contrast, prenatal HIV testing is used to regulate reproductive choices of many poor women as well as women of color.

By and large, when women take an amniocentesis or other prenatal test, they are merely supplied with the results and the significance — that is, the predictive value — of the test. Rarely do these women receive directive counseling strongly urging them to abort. What is most troubling about this contrast is that many of the other prenatal tests have a much higher predictive value of fetal disability than a maternal HIV antibody test. Implicit in the counseling received by HIV-positive women is the judgment that potentially HIV-infected children are less worthy of life than children born with other disabilities.

In those situations where the pregnant woman makes an informed decision to terminate a pregnancy on account of her own HIV infection, it is clearly a good thing that states will fund that abortion under local Medicaid schemes. However, poor women and women of color have learned that reproductive choices are often neither fully informed, nor are they voluntary. As a result, in those states which allow a positive maternal HIV test as a ticket for abortion funding, under circumstances where an abortion is less than voluntary, coerced abortions will become even more commonplace. Indeed, it is foreseeable that as a result of abuses against pregnant women who test HIV-positive, the "right to choose" will no longer mean the right to choose an abortion, but rather the right to choose to carry to term. Again, AIDS turns the issue on its head.

Finally, the implications of forced abortions for HIV-positive women do not take into consideration the various cultural values attached to childbearing. In many communities, a woman's personal and social worth are measured in terms of her ability to bear children. These women, when faced with a 50 to 70 percent chance that a child will not be HIV-infected, may choose to take the risk involved in carrying that pregnancy to term.

AIDS hysteria has halted expansive notions of sexuality, in favor of sexual limitations. Clearly, in this context sex outside certain limited contexts is bad, but particular types of sex will kill you. If this epidemic weren't so tragic, we might find the federal government's campaign of monogamy or abstinence almost silly. A serious response to AIDS invites us to consider alternatives to penile/vaginal methods of sexual expression. However, where this type of real AIDS education has been done, the material has been labeled pornographic, or when in the wrong hands, has resulted in severe penalties for the groups that have developed them.

For example, when graphic and very effective safe sex materials developed by New York City's Gay Men's Health Crisis made their way to the office of Senator Jesse Helms, he promptly used them as a foundation for support of an amendment to a progressive HIV antibody testing and counseling bill. The amendment prohibited federal funding for any organization that promoted or encouraged homosexuality.

Recent sex and sexuality movements have been successful in encouraging each individual to decide what type of sex she or he wishes to have and with whom. AIDS has allowed the government to step back in and define the sexual rules again. By making criminals out of people who engage in certain types of sex, in certain stigmatized contexts, the government is reasserting its authority to set the parameters of legal sex and, by implications, the family. Indeed, some would argue that anything which falls outside these narrow guidelines is not sex at all, but rather an abomination against nature, in the case of sodomy, or a morally repugnant commercial transaction, in the case of prostitution.

The federal government's obsession with monogamy or abstinence as "safe sex" presumes that the only type of sex that people can have is unprotected penile/vaginal intercourse, and that married people are somehow immune from infection. Obviously, this is not true now, nor has it ever been. If anything, we should be talking about sex almost everywhere, with almost everyone in our lives, if we are to begin to permeate the fear, misinformation and prejudice that clouds our understanding of AIDS.

AIDS and AIDS-related infections have had a tremendously damaging effect upon women's sexual expression. In many ways, AIDS has merely magnified the underside of this country. Problems of poor health care, poverty, reproductive abuse, prejudice and bigotry have always existed among us, and AIDS has exacerbated social problems that have never received adequate attention. In so doing, AIDS has taken traditional notions of justice and entitlement and turned them upside down. Public health policies such as prenatal HIV testing are advertised as a shield to protect the health of women who are tested. However, when considered in light of the class, race and ethnicity of many women tested, testing is more of a sword than a shield.

Life And Death: The AIDS Game

SILVIA RAMOS

Silvia Ramos is the executive secretary of the Rio de Janeiro-based Associação Brasileira Interdisciplinar de AIDS (ABIA, Brazilian Interdisciplinary AIDS Association), which carries out studies and research on AIDS and organizes preventive educational campaigns.

BRAZIL IS A country proud of its many records. We have the world's largest river, the planet's largest rain forest, and our country has continental dimensions. One of the most recent records, disclosed by sociologists and political scientists, is the fact that Brazil's economy is the eighth largest of all the capitalist countries (the world's tenth largest), but the salaries of its workers are among the five lowest in the world. This is not an enviable record, but at least it sheds some light on the enormous social, economic and cultural differences between the richest 20 percent and the very poor 80 percent of the Brazilian population.

These very general facts illustrate the situation of a country which has not resolved basic issues such as hunger, food, housing, education and health care for the majority of its people. Therefore, every aspect of large-scale contagious diseases, such as influenza or dengue epidemics, an outbreak of meningitis, or AIDS, becomes a serious problem.

In Brazil, AIDS is not only a public health problem but is, above all, a political problem. Following its tradition of confronting problems only once they have become unsolvable, the Brazilian government is dealing with AIDS in its own peculiar fashion.

Officially only 2,956 AIDS cases had been reported by March 1988; however it is estimated that more than 50 percent of the cases go unreported. Still, the approximately 6,000 cases do not appear to impose a heavy public health danger to a population of 130 million. In relative terms, AIDS is less important than hookworm disease, malaria, yellow fever, and the chronic disease of hunger. Until recently, this justified the laconic response of the public health authorities to all demands for effective action.

This governmental irresponsibility has overlooked the fact that every ten months HIV infection rates have doubled. . .and that if this increase continues, and if something is not done now, there will be at least 6 million cases within the next decade.

In concrete terms, the 500 officially reported AIDS cases in Rio de Janeiro, the country's second largest city, are enough to "stall" the hospital system. There is already a lack of hospital beds, doctors and medication for people with AIDS.

Preventive measures should have started at least four years ago. In February 1988, the government launched a campaign which is both ineffective and dangerous, and is selling fear, the way one sells soap, in little TV spots produced by public relations agencies. These feature dubious slogans such as, "A face can be seen; AIDS can't," and absurd directives such as, "Use condoms in any sexual encounter."

Besides being a political problem, AIDS in Brazil is also a policing problem. The rate of HIV infection through blood transfusions allows our country to claim yet another international record. In Rio de Janeiro, contaminated blood is the cause of about 18 percent of the reported AIDS cases. The blood and blood products trade, as well as the large number of illegal, private and official blood banks which do not test for the HIV antibody, are responsible for this crime.

But what is the social, cultural, sexual and symbolic impact of AIDS on Brazil?

The carnival, the beauty and the swing of the *mulatas*, the beaches of Rio and Bahia, the magic, the charm . . . all these stereotypes not only impress foreign tourists, but in a certain fashion they have also become part of Brazilians' self-image. In that light Brazil could be considered a "sexually liberated" country compared to the antiseptic nature of northern nations.

But contrasting this image, there is a side of Brazil that, deep down, is very conservative. There are profound class and regional differences which make it impossible to speak about a national sexuality. In Brazil — as in those countries with a high number of AIDS cases — AIDS is considered a "gay disease," a result of the "prevailing sexual promiscuity." In some way, the disease has served those who have been anxious to revoke the sexual liberties of recent decades.

Nevertheless, I think that it is still too early to conclude that AIDS has brought or will bring about a victory for the sexual counterrevolution. Along with the epidemic and the prejudice, an equally explosive creativity and solidarity has arisen.

The impact of AIDS on Brazil seems more similar to the North American and European models than to the course that the disease is taking on the African continent and in the Caribbean.

About 95 percent of the reported cases are men. Among those, about 80 percent report homosexual or bisexual experiences. Transmission of the virus due to sexual relations occurred in more than 80 percent of the cases. Unlike Europe and North America, less than 5 percent of the infections were associated with IV drug use. Fourteen percent of the people were infected with contaminated blood and blood products.

While the government estimates that more than 50 percent of the cases go unreported, a number of people think that the percentage is even higher. And more importantly, there is good reason to believe that the largest number of unreported cases is among the poorest people, who might have been infected with contaminated blood. Because they do not belong to any of the classic risk groups, they are not tested for AIDS. They might come to the hospital with pneumonia or another infection and die within a few days. Or they might die at home without medical assistance. If this is correct, the socio-economic-sexual profile of AIDS in Brazil could be, or may become, significantly different from what it is thought to be — a hybrid between what is presently considered to be the African and the European/North American model.

In a recent study carried out by ABIA researchers, the most surprising observations were found in the data on women and AIDS collected by health officials. There seems to be a lot of uncertainty about the facts, and one finds notes like this: "Denies being a prostitute, but the neighbors say she is one." Poor women are classified as "IV drug users — cocaine." IV drug use is quite unusual in Brazil, mostly because the price of such drugs is outrageously high. In terms of the Brazilian AIDS profile, women are a big question mark.

But this is not the case when it comes to the use and abuse of women's image in the official and religious campaigns. The archbishop of Rio de Janeiro recently published an article in a major newspaper, in which he wrote: "I have information that proves that a single prostitute can contaminate 800 men in one year."

Among the 500 cases registered in Rio de Janeiro, there is not one man who was infected through heterosexual intercourse. In contrast, about 35 percent of the women with AIDS were infected heterosexually. There is a clear indication that most women are being infected by bisexual men. The official figures also indicate that 21 percent of the reported cases among women were due to IV drug use, a number that seems quite doubtful. The rest of the cases, about half, are attributed to infection by contaminated blood or are classified as "unknown."

Given that less than 5 percent of the AIDS cases in Brazil are women, it is quite striking that the official prevention campaign is based on a woman's face. Under this face is the slogan: "A face can be seen, AIDS can't." This woman's face appears daily in newspapers, magazines, TV, and on billboards. Images of prostitutes have been used to warn of "the dangers of the night," and the risks of contamination. The image of female prostitution was chosen because she is the most fragile. In Brazil the majority of women who sell their bodies are quite poor, uninformed, and above all, unorganized. There is not one organization in the country to defend the rights of prostitutes.

This is not the case when it comes to gay men.

As we know, prejudice has many faces, one of which is silence. In the official campaigns, male homosexuality was treated in a such a subtle, implicit and timid fashion that the campaigns themselves raise questions. Silence surrounding the transmission of the AIDS virus by gay men is also a subtle and odious form of prejudice. It's irresponsible, if not genocidal.

Maybe the Brazilian government fears possible reactions from gay men's groups who are better organized than prostitutes; or maybe Brazilian machismo does not allow the acknowledgment of widespread homosexual practices prevalent in the big cities. For whatever reason, it is a fact that the image of AIDS projected by the campaign allows the association: woman-prostitute-sexual freedom-sex-death.

Death is a big taboo of occidental societies. From childhood on we are guarded from it. We build our lives denying death, behaving as if we were immortal, as if our existence were infinite. In post-industrial consumer societies, the old is quickly discarded and replaced with the new, and the incessant and irrational production of goods and routines gives meaning to our lives. In such societies, disease, old age and death have to be hidden and preferably forgotten so that we can live. Happily.

In fact, death and disease have been banished from the communities, the neighborhoods, families, and above all, from the home. Today they are lived out at hospitals, removed from our sight, and a good distance away. And sometimes they are even further removed — into intensive care units. The knowledgeable, the technicians and the skilled doctors, treat and administer the bodies of the sick and dying using bureaucratic hospital rituals which allow little interference by the patients or their families. Sometimes these routine treatments include cruel battles against death's arrival. One more week, one more day, one more minute of "life" justifies sacrifices which evoke medieval images of death. Rituals over inert bodies, pierced with tubes, catheters, artificial respirators. . .and arms almost always tied to the small hospital bed, to prevent the dying from freeing themselves of "life," and to finally live their death. In these hospital wars, death, when it finally arrives, is presented like a lost battle, a failure, a mistake, an accident. As if medicine could stop death. . .

But there is something special that happens to death when its existence is denied. Although it has been removed and hidden from our daily lives, it is still there in the form of a diffused and unnamed anxiety — incomprehensible and frightening. It has lost its natural sense and became a senseless occurrence. And, once silenced, it is only spoken of in metaphors.

AIDS is the perfect postmodern metaphor for death. To say the word AIDS is to pronounce a death sentence. I am convinced that a good part of the fiction, irrational fear, panic and prejudices revolving around AIDS are the result of this denial.

For the combination disease-sex-death is triply explosive. It has served to discipline our customs and intimate behavior, and entered like a ghost into this decade, our neighborhoods, our beds. Appearing like a punishment for sexual expression and especially for homosexuality — both of which have been perceived as the spearheads of sexual liberation — it hits full force those who are in the forefront of these recent achievements.

I believe, however, precisely because AIDS unites these strong universal images, it can also be freed from the myths surrounding it. It can be treated within the simple limits of a disease that needs to be prevented and cured, just like any other. And it may also serve to make death and sexuality more visible and to free them from the stereotypes in which they have been imprisoned.

My experience with AIDS has been more determined by pleasures and achievements than by pains and fears. The expressions of solidarity for those who are sick, HIV-positive, and for the support organizations, have been until now more important than the outbursts of prejudice and the creation of fear.

I believe intuitively that AIDS is the symbolic center, the privileged "place" to understand, explain and discover my sexuality. And maybe it is the only space in which to see, to speak and to live daily with the experience of death. In this way, who knows, I can search for my perception of finality and mortality, and thus lead a more intense and liberating life.

VIII

APPENDIX

Glossary of Common AIDS-Related Terms

Acquired Immune Deficiency Syndrome (AIDS) is due to a breakdown of the immune system thought to be caused by the Human Immune Deficiency Virus (HIV). The suppression of the immune system leads to a weakening of the body's defenses against a variety of infections, viruses, fungi and malignancies (cancers). Many of these diseases are called opportunistic since they are a serious threat only for people with deficient immune systems. Some examples of opportunistic diseases associated with AIDS are Pneumocystis carinii pneumonia (PCP), Cytomegalovirus (CMV) and Kaposi's sarcoma (KS).

AIDS symptoms include enlarged lymph nodes, fever and/or night sweats, rapid weight loss and persistent diarrhea. In the United States, an AIDS diagnosis is based on the presence of certain conditions which meet the case definition determined by the Centers for Disease Control (CDC).

In the United States, groups considered to be at high risk for developing AIDS are also officially determined by the CDC. Currently they include gay or bisexual men, IV drug users, hemophiliacs, recipients of transfusions between the years of 1979 and 1985, and the sexual partners of the members of these groups.

AIDS-Related Complex (ARC) is a loose categorization of AIDS-related symptoms which are linked to HIV infection but are not included in the specific case definition of AIDS by the CDC. ARC is not a clearly defined condition and the term is used only in the United States. The differentiation between people with ARC and AIDS is significant because various social services are dependent on an AIDS diagnosis and are not available to people with ARC, even though they might show serious disabling symptoms.

AL-721 is an antiviral drug used to treat AIDS. It is one of several experimental drugs that have shown effects that may be useful in controlling the HIV virus. However, at this time, its effectiveness has not yet been documented.

AZT (Azidothymadine) is an antiviral drug used to treat AIDS. Despite its toxic side effects, it has been known to prolong the lives of some people with AIDS.

Cytomegalovirus (CMV) is a virus in the same family as herpes and chicken pox. While it brings on mild flu symptoms in individuals with normal immune systems, for people with AIDS it can result in severe intestinal, lung or ocular disorders.

ELISA (enzyme-linked immunosorbent assay test) refers to the HIV antibody test which is currently most often used in blood screening programs. Due to its fallibility, the more precise Western blot analysis is usually used to confirm ELISA results.

Hemophilia, a genetic disease that almost exclusively affects men, is a blood coagulation disorder which leads to excessive bleeding. With the development of blood products, such as Factor VIII, the severe effects of this disease have been reduced, although hemophiliacs are still afflicted with certain maladies such as arthritis. At the beginning of 1987, there were about 100 cases of hemophiliacs with AIDS in the United States; a year later there were 534 reported cases. Some researchers are estimating that approximately 35 percent of all hemophiliacs will be diagnosed with AIDS in the next two years.

HIV antibody test involves the examination of an individual's blood for the antibody to the HIV virus. Antibody production is the body's protective response which attempts to counteract the intrusion of foreign substances. Presence of the HIV antibody usually corresponds to infection by the HIV virus. The lag time between a viral infection and the body's production of the corresponding antibody can vary widely. Thus, a person could be recently infected with the HIV virus, but test negative for the corresponding antibody. This test is frequently referred to as the "AIDS test." The most commonly used blood analysis tests for the HIV antibody are ELISA and Western blot.

HIV-positive, HIV-infected and seropositive are all terms to describe a person who has been exposed to and infected with the HIV virus. Many people infected with the HIV virus are healthy and show no AIDS symptoms. It is not yet known what percentage of HIV virus carriers will eventually develop AIDS symptoms. It is believed that everyone carrying the HIV virus may be capable of transmitting it to others through exchange of blood or semen.

Kaposi's sarcoma (KS) is a malignancy associated with AIDS resulting in lesions of the skin, mucous membranes and internal organs. It is uncommon for women with AIDS to develop KS.

Pneumocystis carinii pneumonia (PCP) is a parasitic infection of the lungs which results in persistent fever and bronchial congestion. This is the most common specific infection that meets the case definition for AIDS.

PWA/PWARC are abbreviations for Person(s) with AIDS and Person(s) with ARC.

Seroconversion refers to the development of evidence of antibody in response to an infectious agent. In connection with AIDS, it is used to describe the point at which the HIV antibody can be detected in the blood. It also refers to the process in which infants shed evidence of their mother's immune system and thereby shed the temporary presence of the HIV antibody. Thus it is difficult to accurately determine the HIV status of a newborn.

Seroprevalence refers to the occurrence of a certain blood characteristic within a population. In connection with AIDS it is used to describe the occurrence of individuals who carry the HIV antibody.

STD is an abbreviation for sexually transmitted disease.

T-cells are components of the cellular immune system. T-cell counts are an indication of the body's immune status. However, they are not used as a test for AIDS since many factors such as stress and viral infections can alter the T-cell balance. In HIV-positive people, T-cell counts can be monitored to assess the body's immune status.

Western blot refers to a blood test for the HIV antibody often used as secondary confirmation of an initial positive ELISA antibody test.

AIDS Resources

The following organizations can help you find out more about AIDS-related issues. Some of those frequently mentioned in this book are annotated.

United States

ACT-UP Women's Committee, c/o Maria Maggenti, 337 E 10th St. Apt. 3E, New York, NY 10009, (212) 674-6520.

ADAPT, 85 Bergen St., Brooklyn, NY 11201, (718) 834-9598.

AIDS Action Committee, Women at Risk Group, 661 Boylston St., Boston, MA 02116, (617) 437-6200.

AIDS Homecare and Hospice Program, 225 30th St., San Francisco, CA 94131, (415) 285-5615. Provides an individualized program of professional clinical nursing, social, psychological, spiritual and attendant care in the home for people with AIDS and ARC.

Asian AIDS Project, 2024 Hayes St., San Francisco, CA 94117, (415) 386-4815.

Black Coalition on AIDS, 726 Broderick St., San Francisco, CA 94112, (415) 931-3031.

California Partner's Study, School of Public Health, Epidemiology Program, 140 Warren Hall, UC Berkeley, CA 94720, (415) 642-5512. Provides testing and evaluation, support groups and appropriate referrals for heterosexual partners of PWA/PWARCs, persons who are HIV-positive or persons who have a history of high risk activities. The goal of the study is to research the extent of the HIV infection among heterosexuals and to provide support to partners of HIV-infected individuals.

California Prostitutes Education Project (CAL-PEP), c/o SF AIDS Foundation, P.O. Box 6182, San Francisco, CA 94101-6182, (415) 558-0450. Provides AIDS education for prostitutes and ex-prostitutes. Services include monthly workshops for prostitutes and their lovers, individual counseling, and distribution of condoms and bleach.

Centers for Disease Control (CDC), Atlanta, GA 30333, (404) 329-3311 ext. 3162.

Community Health Project, 208 W 13th St., New York, NY 10011, (212) 675-3559.

Gay American Indians — AIDS Outreach Program, 1347 Divisadero Rm 312, San Francisco, CA 94115, (415) 431-9437.

Gay Men's Health Crisis, 254 W 18th St., New York, NY 10011, (212) 807-6655.

Haitian Coalition on AIDS, 50 Court St. Rm. 605, Brooklyn, NY 11201, (718) 855-7275.

Health Education and Resource Organization (HERO), 101 W. Read St. Rm 819, Baltimore, MD 21201, (301) 685-1180.

Hispanic AIDS Forum, 140 W. 22nd St., New York, NY 10011, (212) 463-8264.

Latino AIDS Project, 2515 24th St., San Francisco, CA 94110, (415) 647-4141.

Lesbian AIDS Project, 25 Belvedere St., San Francisco 94117, (415) 864-8040.

Mid-City Consortium on AIDS, 1779 Haight St., San Francisco, CA 94117, (415) 751-4221. Street-based AIDS education/prevention organization that works specifically with IV drug users.

Minority Task Force on AIDS, 92 St. Nicholas Ave., New York, NY 10026, (212) 749-2816.

Most Holy Redeemer AIDS Support Group, 100 Diamond St., San Francisco, CA 94114, (415) 863-1581.

Mothers of AIDS Patients (MAP), P.O. Box 89049, San Diego, CA 92138, (619) 234-3432 or P.O. Box 1763, Lomita, CA 90717-9998, (213) 450-6485 or (213) 530-2109.

Multicultural Alliance for the Prevention of AIDS (MAPA), 6025 Third St., San Francisco, CA 94124, (415) 822-7500.

National Association of People With AIDS, 1012 14th St. NW, Suite 601, Washington, DC 20005, (202) 347-1317. Promotes self-empowerment of People with AIDS/ARC through education and support.

National Hemophilia Foundation, The Soho Building, 110 Greene St., Rm. 406, New York, NY 10012, (212) 219-8180.

Nicaragua AIDS Education Project, 3181 Mission St., Rm 13, San Francisco, CA 94110.

Open Hand, 1668 Bush St., San Francisco, CA 94109, (415) 771-9808. Provides home delivery meal service seven days a week for people with AIDS/ARC.

People with AIDS Coalition, 263A W 19th St., Rm 125, New York, NY 10011, (212) 627-1810.

Project AWARE, Ward 84, San Francisco General Hospital, 995 Potrero Ave., San Francisco, CA 94110, (415) 476-4091. Conducts AIDS research and health promotion for women in San Francisco at high risk for AIDS via heterosexual transmission. Project AWARE also provides collaborative referral and follow-up for HIV-infected infants of study participants.

San Francisco AIDS Foundation, P.O. Box 6182, San Francisco, CA 94101-6182, (415) 864-4376. Professional AIDS service and advocacy agency providing direct client services in San Francisco and AIDS-related educational services and materials distribution nationwide.

Shanti Project, 525 Howard St., San Francisco, CA 94105-3080, (415) 777-CARE. Provides free volunteer services to people with AIDS and their loved one. Programs include: the Emotional Support Program, the Support Group Program; the Residence Program, the PWA Recreation Program, the PWA Information and Referral Program, and the Speakers Bureau Program.

The Names Project, P.O. Box 14573, San Francisco, CA 94114, (415) 863-5511. A national AIDS memorial quiltpiece and workshop headquartered in San Francisco. The AIDS Quilt is an ongoing project to memorialize people with AIDS who have died.

Women and AIDS Project, 1209 Decater St. NW, Washington, DC 20011.

Women's AIDS Network (WAN), c/o San Francisco AIDS Foundation, P.O. Box 6182, San Francisco, CA 94101-6182, (415) 864-4376 ext. 2030. Provides referrals, advocacy, resource information and support for women affected by AIDS. WAN also develops educational materials and events, and serves as a liaison between other community groups and services related to women and AIDS.

The Women's AIDS Project, 8235 St. Monica Blvd., Suite 201, West Hollywood, CA 90046, (213) 650-1508.

Women's AIDS Resource Network (WARN), 135 W 4th St., New York, NY 10012, (212) 475-6713.

International

AIDS Committee of Toronto, Box 55, Stn F, Toronto, Ont. M4Y 2L4 Canada, (416) 926-1626.

Aids-Hilfe Schweiz, Postfach 1054, CH-8039 Zurich, Switzerland, (01) 201-70-33.

Aids Linien, Knabrostraede 3, 1210 Copenhagen K, Denmark, (01) 91-11-19.

Association AIDES, B.P. 759, 75123 Paris Cedex 03, France, 42-72-19-99.

Association "Vaincre le SIDA," B.P. 435, 75233 Paris Cedex 05, France.

Associazione Solidarieta AIDS (ASA), V. Torricelli 19, 20136 Milano, Italy, 83-94-604.

Berliner Aids-Hilfe, Meinekestr. 12, 1000 Berlin (West) 15, West Germany, 882 5553.

Colectivo de Educacion Popular para la Prevencion del SIDA, Apartado A-262, Managua, Nicaragua.

Empower, P.O. Box 1065, Silom Post Office, Bangkok 10504, Thailand, 234-3078.

GABRIELA — International Affairs Desk, Rm 204, Estuar Bldg., 41 Timog Ave., Quezon City, Philippines.

GAPA, Caixa Postal 04106, CEP 01051 São Paulo/SP, Brazil, (011) 255 5777 ext. 3875.

International Working Group on Women and AIDS, 158 Arlington St., Brighton, MA 02135, USA, (617) 782-1952.

Ministry of Health, P.O. Box 30016, Nairobi, Kenya.

New Zealand AIDS Foundation, Box 6663 Wellesley St., Auckland 1, New Zealand, 33 124.

Österr. Aids-Hilfe, Lenaug. 17, A-1080 Vienna, Austria, (0222) 48-61-86.

Positively Women Group, London, U.K., (01) 291-3120 or (01) 430-2324.

Terrence Higgins Trust Ltd., BM/AIDS, London WC1N 3XX, UK., (01) 833-2971.

The Australian Federation of AIDS organizations, P.O. Box 174, Richmond, Victoria NSW 3121, Australia, 03-417-1759.

Vrouwenplatform en Aids, Maliesingel 46, 3581 B.M., Utrecht, The Netherlands, (030) 312 850.

Women's Action Group, Box 135, Harare, Zimbabwe.

Women's Center, Box 185, Eket, Cross River State, Nigeria.

Selected Bibliography on Women and AIDS

Books

Callen, Michael, ed., *Surviving and Thriving with AIDS, Hints for the Newly-Diagnosed*. New York: People with AIDS Coalition, 1987.

Kübler-Ross, Elisabeth and Mal Warshaw, *AIDS: The Ultimate Challenge*. New York: Macmillan, 1987. Interviews with and reflections on people with AIDS.

Laygues, Hélène, *SIDA témoignage sur la vie et la mort de Martin*. Paris: Hachette, S.A. Editeur (79 blvd. St. Germain, 75006 Paris, France), 1985. The testimony of a woman whose gay business partner/husband died of AIDS.

Moffatt, Bettyclare, *When Someone You Love Has AIDS*. New York: Plume Books, 1987. A book for friends and family.

Moffatt, Bettyclare, et. al., *AIDS: A Self-Care Manual*. Los Angeles: IBS Press/Los Angeles AIDS Project (2339 28th St., Santa Monica, CA 90405, (213) 450-6485), 1987.

Norwood, Chris, *Advice for Life, A Woman's Guide to AIDS Risks and Prevention*. New York: Pantheon Books, 1987. A general handbook.

Panem, Sandra, *The AIDS Bureaucracy*. Cambridge, Mass: Harvard University Press, 1988. A documentation of the U.S. government's failure to deal with the AIDS crisis.

Panos Institute, *AIDS and the Third World*. London: Panos Institute (8 Alfred Place, London WC1E 7EB, UK or 1409 King St., Alexandria, VA 22314, (703) 386-1302), 1988. A valuable dossier outlining statistics on HIV infection and AIDS cases internationally.

Patton, Cindy, *Sex & Germs: The Politics of AIDS*. Boston: South End Press, 1985. A political description of the beginnings of the AIDS epidemic from a gay perspective.

Patton, Cindy and Janis Kelly, *Making It: A Woman's Guide to Sex in the Age of AIDS* (Firebrand Sparks Pamphlet No. 2). Ithaca, NY: Firebrand Books (141 The Commons, Ithaca, NY 14850), 1987. Bilingual (Spanish/English).

Peabody, Barbara, *The Screaming Room, A Mother's Journal of Her Son's Struggle with AIDS*. New York: Avon, 1987.

Pearson, Carol, *Good-Bye, I Love You*. New York: Random House, 1986. A wife describes her gay husband who died of AIDS.

Ralston, Alissa, *What Do Our Children Need to Know About AIDS?*. Novato: Beneficial Publishing (P.O. Box 920, Novato, CA 94948), 1988. Guidelines for parents.

Richardson, Diane, *Women and the AIDS Crisis*. London: Pandora Press, 1987; U.S. edition: *Women and AIDS*, Methuen Inc., 1987. A political handbook, which provides general information. Translated into Dutch and German.

Sabatier, Renée, edit. *Blaming Others: Prejudice, Race and Worldwide AIDS*. Philadelphia: New Society Publishers, 1988.

de Saint Phalle, Niki, *AIDS: You Can't Catch It Holding Hands*. San Francisco: Lapis Press, San Francisco (Box 2010, Novato, CA 94948), 1987. A picture book by the French artist. Recommended for children.

San Francisco AIDS Foundation, *Women and AIDS, A Clinical Resource Guide*, n.d. A collection of articles published in the medical and social service field on women and AIDS.

Walter, Melitta, ed., *Ach wär's doch nur ein böser Traum! Frauen und AIDS*. Freiburg: Kore Verlag (Holbeinstr. 12, D-7800 Freiburg i. Br., West Germany), 1987. An anthology with a variety of theoretical discussions on AIDS issues relevant to women.

Watney, Simon, *Policing Desire: Pornography, AIDS and the Media*. London: Methuen, 1986; U.S. edition: University of Minnesota Press, 1987. A critical look at how the media covers AIDS issues.

Periodicals

The following alternative publications have extensively covered the AIDS epidemic, including articles by and about women.

Body Positive, 263A W. 19th St. Rm. 107, New York, NY 10011. A monthly for HIV-positive people.

Coming Up! 592 Castro St., San Francisco, CA 94114.

Gay Community News, 62 Berkeley, Boston, MA 02116. Lesbian and gay weekly.

Newsline, PWA Coalition, 236A West 19th St., Rm. 125, New York, NY 10011. A monthly for people with AIDS.

Radical America, 1 Summer St., Somerville, MA 02143. "Facing AIDS," special issue (Vol. 20, No. 6, Nov-Dec. 1986).

Rites, P.O. Box 65, Station F, Toronto, Ontario M4Y 2L4, Canada. Gay and lesbian monthly.

San Francisco Sentinel, 500 Hayes St., San Francisco, CA 94102.

The New Internationalist, 175 Carlton St., Toronto, Ontario M5A 2K3, Canada; or 42 Hythe Bridge St., Oxford OX1 2EP, UK; or P.O. Box 82, Fitzroy, Victoria 3065, Australia. "The Politics of AIDS," special issue, March 1987.

The Village Voice, 842 Broadway, New York, NY 10003. New York weekly.

Films and Videos

Among the many films and videos produced on AIDS issues, we suggest the following:

"AIDS and the Women's Community," co-produced by the San Francisco AIDS Foundation and Bay Area Career Women. An in-depth view of the AIDS epidemic's critical impact on the lesbian community.

"Dying for Love, The Impact of AIDS on the American Woman," Lifetime Cabletelevision Network, 1211 Avenue of the Americas, New York, NY 10036. TV documentary recounting the trauma and isolation of women living with AIDS.

"Ojos Que No Ven" ("Eyes That Fail to See"), Instituto Familiar De La Raza and Adinfinitum Films. An AIDS education tool for Spanish speakers. Ojos presents a culturally appropriate treatment of teenage sexuality, homosexuality, IV drug use, and prostitution.

"Too Little, Too Late," a documentary by Micki Dickoff, Fanlight Production. Focusing on the biological families of PWAs. With Barbara Peabody and Miriam Thompson, founders of Mothers of AIDS Patients (MAP).

"Women, Children and AIDS: Researchers' Perspectives," produced by Jane Wagner. A documentary on the goals and findings of a California-based research project studying women and children with AIDS, ARC or at high-risk.

About the Editors

Ines Rieder was born in Vienna in 1954. She has studied political science, anthropology, and social work, and works as free-lance writer and translator. Active in the international women's movement since the 1970s, she has worked with the Oakland-based People's Translation Service, publisher of *Newsfront International*. She was a member of the collective which produced *Second Class, Working Class*, an international feminist reader, and was one of the founders of *Connexions*, an international women's quarterly. After taking care of her friend Michael, who died of AIDS in Paris in June 1986, she started researching and writing on international AIDS issues, focussing on women's roles in dealing with and covering the epidemic.

Patricia Ruppelt was born in Long Beach in 1956 and lives in Oakland, CA. Involved with women's publishing since 1979, she was a collective member of *Connexions* for five years. She attended and reported on the NGO Women's Forum and UN Women's Conference in Nairobi, Kenya in 1985. For the last year, she has been a member of the San Francisco Women's AIDS Network. Over the past eleven years, she has traveled extensively in South and Southeast Asia. The particular focus of her travels has been women's organizations in these countries, especially in India.